Medical
MARIJUANA
101

MEDICAL MARIJUANA 101
Copyright © 2011 Mickey Martin and Ed Rosenthal

Published by Quick American Publishing
A division of Quick Trading Co.
Oakland, California

ISBN 13: 978-0-932551-93-1
Printed in U.S.A.

Project Managers: Jane Klein and Nick Rosenthal
Cover: Hera Lee
Interior Design and Layout: Alvaro Villanueva
Editing: Eva Saelens
Editorial Advisors: DJ Sun and Mary Lynn Mathre, R.N.

Publisher's Cataloging-in-Publication
(Provided by Quality Books, Inc.)

    Martin, Mickey, 1974-
       Medical marijuana 101 / by Mickey Martin with
    Ed Rosenthal, Gregory T. Carter, M.D.
       p. cm.
       Includes bibliographical references.
       ISBN-13: 978-0-932551-93-1
       ISBN-10: 0-932551-93-9
       ISBN-13: 978-1-936807-15-4
       ISBN-10: 1-936807-15-7

       1. Marijuana--Therapeutic use. 2. Cannabis--
    Therapeutic use.   I. Rosenthal, Ed. II. Carter,
    Gregory T. III. Title.

    RM666.C266M37 2011   615.7'827
             QBI11-600200

Medical
MARIJUANA
101

by Mickey Martin
with Ed Rosenthal and Gregory T. Carter, M.D.

WITHDRAWN

QUICK
AMERICAN

Harborside Health Center in Oakland, CA offers a wide variety of strains that are labeled regarding qualities and potency.

URPLE C

DREAM QUEEN
(I/S)

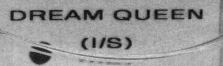

MANGO OG

(I/S)

19.7%
THC

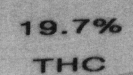

PYREX®

CONTENTS

Foreword

In 2000, I sustained a severe neck injury that left me with lack of mobility in my neck, neurological spasms, and severe chronic pain. I had to take painkillers, muscle relaxants, and high doses of ibuprofen to relieve the pain and calm the spasms. After about a year, as a result of the medications, problems developed with my stomach and kidneys. Six months later, my doctor warned me that I might have to start dialysis. I was 23 years old and terrified.

One day in the examining room, my doctor shut the door behind him and asked me in a whisper, "Do you smoke marijuana?" I said no, and he replied, "Do you know anyone who does?" I thought he was trying to buy marijuana from me! My doctor reassured me that my assumption was wrong. He explained that he did not know very much about medical cannabis, but he had had other patients with similar intolerance to pain medications who were able to cut their medication intake by at least half by using cannabis. He was reluctant to put me on dialysis. If I could find some marijuana, we should try it.

It was the first time that I had ever really thought about marijuana as medicine. I probably had the same amount of information on the subject that most Americans had at the time. I thought medical cannabis was only for people with AIDS or cancer. In favor of it in principle, I knew little about the emerging scientific developments nor had considered the needs of patients. Now facing my own medical crisis, the choice between dialysis and cannabis seemed an easy one to make, regardless of the law.

Finding information about cannabis as medicine was extremely difficult. I started by calling friends and friends of friends, but none of these individuals could explain how to use cannabis as a medicine and why cannabis worked. I felt alone as I started experimenting. It wasn't until months later when I could visit the medical cannabis centers in California's San Francisco Bay Area that I was able to get the kinds of information found in this book.

Access Means Action

So much has changed over the past years. Resources like this book make learning about cannabis therapeutics and policies easier for patients. But indisputably the battle for safe and legal access to this medication rages on.

The history of medical cannabis in the U.S. is filled with stories of the heroic patients who had laid the foundation of safe access. At the heart of this movement are individuals willing to commit daily acts of federal civil disobedience to provide medicine to people like me—a movement of people willing to stand up against injustice, people willing to fight in the courtroom, and people willing to spend their last days concerned about the welfare of others.

I decided to work with other medical cannabis stakeholders to create an organization that would stand up for the rights of people like me who were seeking safe access, as well as the rights of those willing to provide it. As a cannabis patient, it was my turn, my responsibility, and my honor.

In 2002 the opportunity came to found and direct Americans for Safe Access, ASA, the first organization dedicated to safe and legal access to cannabis (marijuana) for therapeutic uses and research.

ASA created a vision for what safe access should look like, and the legal framework to support that vision, through the passing of state and local laws and numerous court battles. Our extensive monitoring of law enforcement activity has helped thousands of patients, and held law enforcement accountable to state laws. We continue to work with members of Congress and the Administration to resolve the federal conflict.

By even considering cannabis as your choice of medicine, you are formulating the future of medical cannabis in your city, state, and nation. My hope is that as you discover the utility of cannabis as a therapeutic in your life, you will also join in to guarantee safe and legal access for everyone who needs it.

Sincerely,

STEPH SHERER
Founder and Executive Director
Americans for Safe Access

Chapter 1

Introduction

Unexpected and unplanned-for ailments arise in life, no matter how healthy a person's lifestyle. Imagine waking in the night to shooting pain and uncontrollable spasms in your legs, only to discover it is the beginning stages of multiple sclerosis (MS). What if you begin to experience severe abdominal pain and your physician diagnoses you with Crohn's disease? Alternatively, what if you survive a serious auto accident only to be left with a permanent pain in your legs?

Additionally, less serious but still troublesome health problems become issues for everyone at some point in their lives. Glaucoma, arthritis, migraine headaches, and depression are all examples of extremely common, usually non-life-threatening, health problems that often occur spontaneously and without explanation.

> Unfortunately, you're left to choose between feeling better and breaking the law.

Now suppose you realize that the most effective treatment for your disorder is marijuana? Unfortunately, you're left to choose between feeling better and breaking the law. You may have been taught that only degenerates and delinquents use illegal drugs. Now you found an illegal drug that eases your pain and suffering. What will you do? You may be hesitant about trying it for your own condition. After all, it is not available in regular pharmacies and there is so much controversy surrounding it. In addition there may be legal implications.

Medical Marijuana 101 explores the science and history of the marijuana plant and provides a solid foundation to form an educated decision about whether you could benefit from this medicine.

> Humans have used marijuana therapeutically for thousands of years.

Humans have used marijuana therapeutically for thousands of years because the herb controls or alleviates a wide variety of medical symptoms. We'll explore the science of how marijuana works and its medical uses and effects. We'll also examine its history, how it's produced and the politics, economics, and legality of marijuana.

What is marijuana?

Marijuana is a flowering plant with many different varieties sharing many chemical characteristics. However the varieties have different effects that provide targeted benefits for a wide range of medical conditions. Marijuana is a hearty plant that adapted to many different climates and growing conditions. You may be familiar with the common image of the five-fingered marijuana leaf. These leaves grow along strong branches that extend laterally from the main stem. The flowers develop along the ends of the branches, forming thick clusters that are usually thin and long or bulky. They produce a sticky crystalline resin and have a strong, sweet-to-pungent aroma. Some varieties grow tall and lanky, while others grow short and bushy. Each variety has its own growth rate, appearance, and medical usefulness.

The term "buds" refers to the dried flowers of the female plant. Buds contain the medicinal compounds and are the part of the plant that is typically used. The leaves are used to make extracts because they contain small quantities of the active ingredients found in marijuana.

Can you ignore the societal stigma
attached to this simple plant?

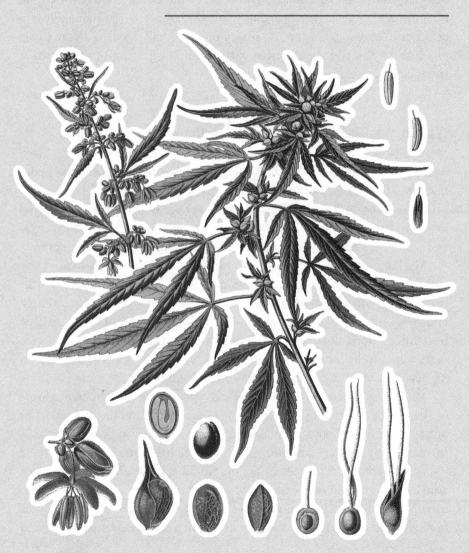

Marijuana is different from other annual plants because it is "dioecious," meaning male and female flowers grow on separate plants. When the female plants are not pollinated the flowers remain seedless. These seedless buds are known as "sinsemilla," Spanish for "without seed". These sinsemilla buds are distributed in medical marijuana dispensaries. Marijuana growers select only female plants so the plants produce only seedless buds. Chapters 7 and 8 describe the different varieties of marijuana and the basics of marijuana horticulture

Why is marijuana an effective medicine?

Marijuana has beneficial uses for many medical conditions. You may have heard jokes about the "munchies," slang term for the increase in appetite that often follows use of marijuana. For many sick people, appetite stimulation is an important step toward wellness. Proper nourishment is required for us to be healthy, so a substance that increases appetite and eating is essential to the recovery of patients who suffer from anorexia, for example.

Marijuana reduces nausea and vomiting, which often accompanies chemotherapy. Cannabis eliminates the nauseous, sick-to-the-stomach feeling and prevents vomiting, which is violent and physically taxing. Nausea and vomiting lead to dehydration and weight loss, extending recovery time because the body doesn't retain enough nutrients to heal properly. Since marijuana can be inhaled or used as a tincture, it is more effective against nausea than ingesting a pill, which is often regurgitated.

Marijuana is an effective pain reliever, especially in cases of neuropathic or "burning and shooting" types of pain. The anti-inflammatory properties of the active ingredients of the marijuana plant have also proven useful in treating many medical conditions including arthritis and glaucoma.

One of the most important factors in choosing marijuana as a medicine is its safety. There are no fatalities from marijuana and an overdose usually leads to a desire to lay down and go to sleep. In comparison, many prescription and over-the-counter pain medicines are extremely toxic and addictive. Marijuana provides a natural alternative to some of these dangers with comparatively low addictive potential.

How does marijuana affect these symptoms? The simple explanation is your body responds to the active ingredients of marijuana, known as cannabinoids, much like it responds to your body's own naturally produced endocannabinoids. Endocannabinoids are found in the brains and bodies of all animals except insects and have evolved over millions of years. The effects of the active ingredients of the marijuana plant, the cannabinoids, mirror the effects of our own internal endocannabinoids. We'll explore specifically how marijuana creates beneficial and palliative effects on physically debilitating symptoms in Chapter 3.

When I'm asked, "Why is marijuana an effective medicine?" I usually answer, "Because it works." It is a natural plant substance that can be as effective, or in some cases more effective, than many commonly prescribed, side effect loaded synthetic drugs. As with any medication, always consult your physician before using marijuana to replace any medicine or to confirm its safety when taken in conjunction with other medications.

How do you know marijuana is safe?

Because of the decades of misinformation about the perceived dangers of marijuana, people often question its safety as a medicine. The undeniable truth is marijuana is extremely safe. Consider this: Marijuana has never caused a single recorded fatal overdose.

Animal studies have shown that a lethal dose of cannabinoids would be in the neighborhood of 40,000 times the typical human dose. This would be like in taking 40 to 80 pounds of marijuana buds or their extracts all at once. This amount is impossible to consume, so death is not a risk when using marijuana. You don't need to worry about dying from an overdose of marijuana unless you plan to smoke a telephone-pole-sized joint in 10 minutes or less.

There are certain dangers related to using marijuana. Patients report adverse effects such as feeling overwhelmed, panicked, paranoid, or experiencing an increased heart rate. Some strains, especially those with extremely high THC content, are more likely to affect new patients in these ways. Strains with high CBD content modulate the effects of THC, so they are less likely to have these adverse affects. Sometimes it's unclear a complaint relates to an adverse reaction or if it is due to the patient's mental state.

Many people have deep-seated fears about using marijuana because of the criminality associated with it. This fear alone can raise your heartbeat. As with many medicines, marijuana affects everybody a bit differently. Marijuana is not a good option for some people, just as with all medicines.

Another potential concern when considering marijuana as medicine is that it is an herb, and if you did not grow it yourself you don't know how it was grown. Unhygienic practices, such as the use of chemical pesticides, leave harsh residues on the plant that are dangerous to ingest or inhale. Molds and fungus also pose a risk to some patients. For these reasons it's best to know where your medicine is coming from. Chapter 4 discusses these issues in more detail.

Any substance can be unsafe if used incorrectly or abused and marijuana is no different. Its effect on some users make them incapable of driving a car, operating machinery, or executing other tasks that require a high level of concentration. Marijuana should always be used in a responsible and controlled setting. If you adhere to basic safety protocols and manage your dosage effectively, you will have a completely safe experience.

Why then is marijuana illegal?

In 1937, the Marihuana Stamp Tax Act made the commercial cultivation, distribution, and use of marijuana and hemp products illegal in the United States without first obtaining a government-issued tax stamp. Since the authorities issued very few stamps, the Stamp Tax Act effectively outlawed marijuana. Thirty-three years later Congress passed the Controlled Substances Act (CSA), enacted into law as Title II of the Comprehensive Drug

Abuse Prevention and Control Act of 1970. The CSA, among other things, created legislation surrounding banned drugs including marijuana and commissioned the Drug Enforcement and Food and Drug Administrations (DEA and FDA) to create "schedules" to classify all drugs. Marijuana was classified a Schedule I substance, which is described as a drug with "a high abuse potential and no currently accepted medical use in treatment in the United States, and a lack of accepted safety for use of the drug or other substance under medical supervision." This classification, which places marijuana in the same category as heroin and a long list of other opiates is incorrect and unjust. Marijuana has a myriad number of medical applications and despite overwhelming evidence to the contrary, federal lawmakers do not yet recognize the therapeutic values of marijuana.

Some states have passed legislation permitting medical use of marijuana under controlled circumstances. The situation is fluid and more states are passing ballot initiatives and enacting legislation to legalize and or decriminalize the medical use of marijuana. Many states have enacted laws to set up and regulate marijuana distribution systems for patients to access marijuana as a prescribed medicine. It is your responsibility as a patient

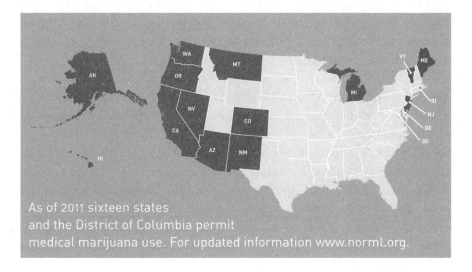

As of 2011 sixteen states and the District of Columbia permit medical marijuana use. For updated information www.norml.org.

to know the laws that govern the medical use of marijuana in your area—courts in a state that does not recognize medical marijuana will probably not be sympathetic if you are arrested for marijuana possession and claim it was for medicinal purposes.

As time goes on and more people demand safe access to medical marijuana, it will be increasingly difficult for the federal government to continue the criminalization of its medical use. Additionally, in every election cycle new states legalize it, which puts more pressure on the federal government to loosen the prohibition of marijuana.

One might reasonably conclude that marijuana's illegality is clearly a mistake. Yet an unwise law is a law nonetheless, and all medical marijuana users must act with caution when obtaining and using their medicine. Chapter 9 addresses your legal rights as a medical marijuana patient.

What do doctors say about medical marijuana?

Many doctors agree that marijuana possesses viable medicinal properties, but because many other doctors are unaware of current medicinal marijuana studies, they hesitate to recommend it as medicine, even where it is legal. Increasingly, however, doctors and organizations are recognizing the therapeutic medical benefits of marijuana in the face of experience and a growing body of research.

In fact, most major medical organizations, including the American Medical Association (AMA) and the American College of Physicians (ACP), endorse the rescheduling of marijuana to reflect its medicinal properties and to open the door to further research. The American Public Health Association (1995) and the American Nurses Association (2003) are also both strong supporters of patient access to marijuana.

The ACP stated, "[We] urge review of marijuana's status as a Schedule I controlled substance and reclassification into a more appropriate schedule, given the scientific evidence regarding marijuana's safety and efficacy in some clinical conditions. ... Given marijuana's proven efficacy at treating certain symptoms and its relatively low toxicity, reclassification would reduce barriers to research and increase availability of cannabinoid drugs to patients who have failed to respond to other treatments."

The AMA adopted the report "Use of Marijuana for Medicinal Purposes" from the Council on Science and Public Health (CSAPH). The report affirms marijuana has medicinal values and calls for expanded research in this area. It concludes "short term controlled trials indicate that smoked cannabis reduces neuropathic pain, improves appetite, and caloric intake especially in patients with reduced muscle mass, and may relieve spasticity and pain in patients with multiple sclerosis." In 2010, the AMA called for a review of the Schedule I status of cannabis in order to advance its use as a medicine.

For a current list of supporting organizations including health care professionals, visit the Patients Out of Time Web site, a totally volunteer organization, at www.MedicalMarijuana.com. There are hundreds on their current list. If your doctor is uninformed or has a knee-jerk response to your questions, seek out a doctor more familiar with marijuana therapies before deciding if it is right for you.

Is there credible research on marijuana as a medicine?

Yes. Reliable studies have been conducted to determine the efficacy of marijuana as a medicine. In the United States only a few institutions have been allowed to pursue research, because of the Schedule I status of the plant. The results of studies at one of these institutions, the Center for Medical Marijuana Research at the University of California San Diego, found it to be an effective treatment for pain and spasms associated with multiple sclerosis and other neurological afflictions. In Canada the McGill University Health Centre reported similar results in a study published in the *Canadian Medical Association Journal*. The study confirmed that people suffering from chronic neuropathic pain from nerve injury found relief by using controlled dosages of smoked marijuana. They also reported improved moods and better sleep. Both studies validated that low doses of the cannabinoid THC provided good results with minimal psychoactive side effects.

Over 6,500 peer reviewed reports in international medical journals confirm marijuana's medicinal value. These publications addressed the various effects of marijuana use including its capacity to retard cancer cell growth, its ability to alleviate the pain and nausea of chemotherapy, and the effectiveness of different delivery methods. Some clinical studies have been disregarded as invalid because they were not sanctioned FDA-approved clinical studies. However, the U.S. federal government has long stifled any significant amounts of "approved" research in this field. One way the government impedes research is by controlling the supply of marijuana used in these studies.

It is virtually impossible to pursue research into marijuana because of the circular and nonsensical rules imposed by the U.S. government. To be allowed to do marijuana research, one must have a government grant; to get a government grant, one must do pilot research; to do pilot research, one must have marijuana; to get marijuana in the laboratory, one must have a government grant.

Researchers and institutions must have the proper Schedule I accreditations to be allowed even to possess such "dangerous compounds," and the DEA regulates such licensure with an equally restrictive attitude. Researchers face one final challenge: The marijuana provided by the U.S. government for research is clearly of lesser quality and potency than the marijuana commonly available from public dispensaries for legal medicinal use. The consistency of the samples and the strains also affects the outcome of the research. These hurdles make the federal government's position quite clear regarding its overall concern for legitimate medicinal marijuana research: It doesn't want to discover or distribute the truth.

Still, a large body of peer-reviewed controlled studies indicate the great potential for medicinal marijuana. Only when the stranglehold on marijuana research is ended will researchers be free to explore all its potential medical benefits.

How do I know if marijuana is a good medicine for me?

Maybe you've tried marijuana in the past but never really considered its medicinal qualities. Or maybe you've never tried marijuana. The first issue to consider is medical need. Do you have a condition that use of marijuana might benefit? Chapter 3 considers specific conditions for which marijuana can be helpful.

Always discuss whether marijuana is a good choice with a trusted medical professional. Be aware of local laws and learn about the drug testing regimen used by employers. Because marijuana is reemerging into society as a legitimate medicine, it is less taboo than it once was, but there are still social and cultural factors that may affect your decision. Friends' and family's concerns and misunderstandings can be overcome with basic education, but you still may experience skepticism from people who have spent their lifetimes hearing that marijuana is a "dangerous," "illicit" drug only used by felons and reprobates. It is your decision to make, and ultimately it is your health at stake.

Your decision may be influenced by the knowledge that many people find great relief from this natural and powerful plant. Don't decide hastily or under pressure. If marijuana makes you feel better chances are it is a good choice for you. If it is does not contribute to your well being, however, or if you experience adverse effects when using it, it is obviously not a good option for you. If using marijuana will cause you to lose your job or alienate your loved ones, it's obviously not a good alternative for you. Only you can answer these questions and make the best decision for your situation.

> It is your decision to make, and ultimately it is your health at stake.

Chapter 2

The Medical Effects of Marijuana and the Science Behind It

Why does marijuana make you feel better? Marijuana contains hundreds of natural chemical compounds, many of which possess psychoactive and therapeutic properties that work within your body to produce positive effects that support healing. Whether you inhale or ingest marijuana, its active ingredients make their way to your blood stream and interact with your body to produce beneficial effects. The chemical compounds that make marijuana an effective medication are called cannabinoids.

What is a cannabinoid?

You've heard the term THC in reference to marijuana. THC is short for delta-9-tetrahydrocannabinol, the most prominent psychoactive cannabinoid found in marijuana. Cannabinoids are pharmacologically active compounds. THC is one of them. When you use marijuana, the cannabinoids find their way to their target, your body's cannabinoid receptors. The cannabinoids bind to one of the receptors. This might make you feel euphoric and relieves the symptoms of your medical condition.

THE CANNABINOIDS

The major active chemical compounds found in marijuana are:

- DELTA-9-TETRAHYDROCANNABINOL (Δ9-THC): THC is the most psychoactive cannabinoid found in marijuana. THCA (tetrahydrocannabinolic acid) is highly concentrated in the flowering clusters or buds. It converts to the more active form, THC, as it dries.

- CANNABIDOL (CBD): CBD is the second most predominant cannabinoid in marijuana. This compound continues to provoke interest for its therapeutic value. It has little or no psychoactive properties. Researchers and patients have begun to focus on the beneficial effects of using THC and CBD together, as well as on CBD's individual effect on diseases and afflictions. CBD reduces anxiety and panic in some patients. It is an anti-inflammatory, sedative, and a neuroprotective agent. Medical demand is high for CBD-rich strains so marijuana breeders have begun to producing high CBD levels plants. Entire websites (such as www.ProjectCBD.org) are dedicated to the understanding of this cannabinoid and its positive effects on human health.

- CANNABIGEROLIC ACID: a chemical precursor to THC and CBD

- CANNABINOL (CBN): The third most prevalent chemical compound in marijuana, cannabinol is the incidental product of the chemical breakdown of THC. You may find higher levels of CBN in improperly stored marijuana resulting in weakened, diminished medical effect.

How does your body process marijuana?

The effects of marijuana are produced by a cannabinoid receptor system in your body consisting of at least two receptor types: CB1 and CB2. CB1 receptors are found exclusively in the brain. They are concentrated in the hippocampus and cerebral cortex (see illustration on p. 16), which control memory and cognition. CB1 receptors interact with marijuana's active com-

- ⊙ TERPENOIDS: These plant-produced odor molecules result in marijuana's distinct aroma. They affect the quality of the experience by altering THC's effects. They determine whether the effect is relaxing, energizing or bubbly. The terpenoids alter the effects of the cannabinoids pharmacologically.

- ⊙ FLAVONOIDS: Marijuana has over 20 known flavonoids, a large class of water-soluble plant pigments that contribute to plant color. Marijuana has unique flavonoids—dubbed cannaflavins—that have both anti-inflammatory and antioxidant properties. Flavonoids may immobilize viruses and allergens. Studies have demonstrated their carcinogenic properties as well.

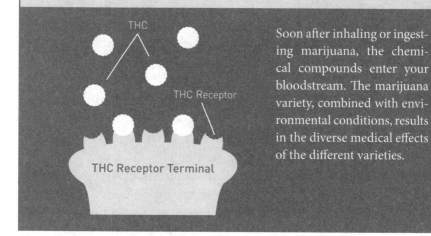

Soon after inhaling or ingesting marijuana, the chemical compounds enter your bloodstream. The marijuana variety, combined with environmental conditions, results in the diverse medical effects of the different varieties.

pounds to produce its psychoactive effects including the euphoric, blissful state that often makes pain more manageable.

CB2 receptors are termed "peripheral receptors" because they are found outside the brain, primarily in the immune system and organs, especially the spleen and in white blood cells. They may be responsible for the cannabinoids' other effects, including the reduction of inflammation. Some

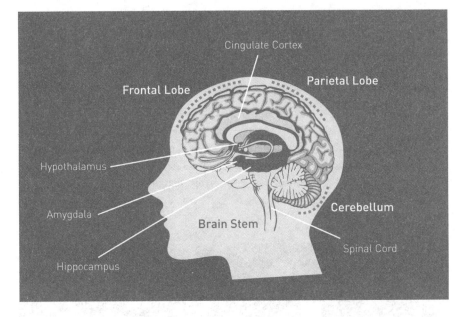

The cannabinoid receptor system is where marijuana becomes medicine.

studies indicate beneficial effects from marijuana on neurodegenerative disorders such as Alzheimer's, Parkinson's, and Huntington's diseases.

The cannabinoid receptor system is where marijuana becomes medicine. These receptors enable humans to obtain the beneficial effects of marijuana's active ingredients. They regulate numerous biological actions within your body including learning, memory, motor skills, pain relief, body temperature, and heart rate. It is used medically to suppress nausea and alleviate pressure in the eye.

What is an endocannabinoid?

Endocannabinoids are substances produced naturally by your body that activate the CB1 and CB2 receptors to regulate body processes and provide relief from stress and discomfort. The principal endocannabinoid is arachidonylethanolamide, or anandamide (AEA). This naturally occurring lipid is a neurotransmitter found in the brains of all animals on the planet except insects. Researchers are working to find the correlation between AEA and human memory, eating habits, sleep patterns, and pain relief. Studies in rats show that it regulates hunger and food intake.

The name anandamide is derived from the Sanskrit word for bliss, *ananda*.

The endocannabinoid system has multiple functions including regulating immunity, inflammation, neurotoxicity, blood pressure, appetite, gastrointestinal function, glaucoma, epilepsy, depression, and stress. It helps regulate the body's biological responses to maintain health and activity by restoring balance. There is no human physiological system yet investigated that is not modulated by the endocannabinoid system.

How will marijuana make you feel?

Usually pretty good. Marijuana creates an intense feeling of well-being. But it doesn't make everyone feel good all of the time; just most people, most of the time. Your tolerance to it, its potency, and method of intake all affect the intensity that marijuana has on your mind and body.

Inhaling marijuana is the quickest route to the brain. It has a much more rapid onset than when ingesting it in food since it must be digested before its effects are felt. When you inhale, your biological responses change almost instantly. You may find that your throat is dry or that you are thirsty. Your eyes become a little red due to dilation of the blood vessels of the eye. You may look drowsy, an effect called "pseudopodia," when the musculature of your eyes become relaxed. If you're a glaucoma patient or suffer from tension afflictions, you may find the pressure reduced in and around your eyes. Your heart may begin to race a little bit, increasing blood flow throughout your body. The upper bronchial passages of your lungs may expand. You'll most likely feel a relaxing sensation come over you and in a short time you will likely become hungry.

Relaxation, reduced tension, thirst, and hunger are the effects experienced by a majority of people. Some report a comparatively minimal effect during their first few experiences with marijuana, so you may want to try it a couple of times to ensure you are experiencing the total effect. It may take your body chemistry some time to adapt to the biological changes. For this reason, it's best not to rapidly increase your dosage during your first marijuana experiences. It is better to increase the dosage gradually over several experiences if necessary.

Some people don't react well to marijuana and report a feeling of anxiety, panic, and dizziness. Anxieties induced by marijuana can create an unpleasant experience. A person under this type of duress will not experience marijuana's therapeutic value. If you experience a response to marijuana intake that induces anxiety, reducing the dosage for your next exposure might be warranted or perhaps marijuana simply isn't the right medication for you.

Another consideration is that there are many strains of marijuana. Each has its own chemical composition. One may produce a more desirable effect than another. The method of administration can also make a difference. Marijuana can be administered in a number of ways. These are discussed in detail in Chapter 6. If you experience a negative reaction, don't panic. Marijuana is safe and nontoxic. Depending on how much marijuana you take in, the symptoms will almost always go away within a few hours.

DON'T BELIEVE THE HYPE.
COMMON MYTHS ABOUT MARIJUANA DEBUNKED

Marijuana has a bad rap. Decades of prohibition have left us uneducated, even scared, of marijuana. Unfortunately, this relatively benign plant is demonized and associated with the lazy, derelict, and criminal fringe of society. Here are some common, though erroneous, claims made about the people who use marijuana:

MARIJUANA MAKES YOU STUPID: This is at the core of the language used to describe a "stoner" or marijuana user. The myth that marijuana kills brain cells or causes brain damage has absolutely no basis in fact. The "stupid" theory also covers the claim that marijuana diminishes your memory.

Most of the misinformation came from one often-cited study performed on monkeys that was later fully disproved by studies on humans in Jamaica and Costa Rica by the U.S. National Center for Toxicological Research and SRI International. Studies on humans found almost no perceivable knowledge deficiency from marijuana use in humans, even after very heavy use.

Like other mind-altering medications, marijuana might temporarily affect your ability to recall facts, verbalize thoughts, concentrate, or learn effectively. These effects normally subside as the medicine wears off, but heavy users may experience more lasting effects. Within a short time all effects go away.

MARIJUANA MAKES YOU LAZY: Marijuana use is often associated with laziness or a lack of motivation in users. While some varieties of marijuana do have a sedative effect and can even cause extreme relaxation, studies have disproven the myth. Many successful, motivated, ambitious people use marijuana regularly.

Most people who use marijuana as a medicine do not experience lack of motivation and ambition. On the contrary, marijuana often serves to ease a patient's medical symptoms, which are the real "anti-motivators" in their lives. Their increased physical well-being allows them to live more full and active lives.

MARIJUANA LIMITS YOUR ABILITY TO HAVE CHILDREN: One of the biggest myths about marijuana is that it makes men sterile or impairs reproductive ability. There is no single confirmed case of impaired fertility due to marijuana use. There is no research to confirm lowered sex hormones in men or women who use marijuana. The National Institute on Drug Abuse states that marijuana has no permanent effect on human reproductive systems.

MARIJUANA LEADS TO USING HARD DRUGS: This is known as the "gateway drug" theory. There is no scientific basis to this theory. Marijuana has not been shown to lead to the use of harder drugs like cocaine or heroin. No substance or combination of substances in marijuana has been shown to program the brain to desire harder drugs.

This "gateway" claim is often made on the assumption that a person tries marijuana first before moving on to other drugs. In countries such as the Netherlands and Portugal, where marijuana is accepted and legalized, there are not elevated abuse rates for illicit drugs. Quite to the contrary, when these countries ended marijuana prohibition, teenage use declined, likely because the drug was no longer considered taboo. However, because of marijuana's illegal status elsewhere, people may be exposed to the illicit drug market.

MARIJUANA MAKES PEOPLE VIOLENT: This fallacy began in the early twentieth century to demonize marijuana users and create fear about its use. If anything, the exact opposite is true. Marijuana's temporary sedative effects usually makes people temporarily passive, laid-back, and relaxed. All claims that marijuana makes people violent have been firmly rejected by scientific studies including a report by the National Academy of Sciences that concludes, "…studies in human beings have failed to yield evidence that marijuana use leads to increased aggression."

Some Real Dangers

Marijuana is not completely free from dangers or concerns. Even though most patients report the benefits of marijuana use far outweigh the inherent negatives, there are two real considerations to reflect on when using marijuana: the effect of smoking on your long-term health and dangers that may arise during temporary mental impairment. The good news is both concerns can be greatly reduced by using a little common sense.

You can avoid the negative side effects of smoking by using alternative delivery methods such as a vaporization device, adding marijuana oils, tinctures, or extracts into food or drinks, or adding them to topical ointments. Vaporizers heat marijuana to a temperature that effectively vaporizes the active ingredients without burning away most of the plant matter. Vaporizing, using tinctures, and ingesting marijuana eliminate the smoke. Chapter 6 explains alternatives to inhaling in detail.

When you are affected by marijuana your motor skills and ability to accomplish certain tasks may decrease and the likelihood of having an accident may increase. Do not drive a car, operate heavy machinery, or perform tasks that require a great deal of concentration while under the influence of marijuana.

Numerous studies show that impairment from marijuana is far less profound and less dangerous than alcohol impairment, but the dangers are real. Marijuana's effects are strongest during the first couple of hours after intake and absorption. With regular use many patients develop a tolerance to its psychoactive effects and are not as impaired. To be safe, err on the side of caution and never put yourself in danger by using marijuana in potentially dangerous situations.

> To be safe, always err on the side of caution and never put yourself in danger by using marijuana in potentially dangerous situations.

Is Marijuana a Good Choice for You?

We are each responsible for our own well-being. The first step in deciding if marijuana may be a viable medicine for you is to assess your need. What condition do you suffer from and how can marijuana alleviate your symptoms? Chapter 3 explores the many conditions and symptoms marijuana can help. Like many medicines it may be a matter of trial and error before you find the best strain of marijuana and the best intake method. Only you can really know if marijuana makes you feel better. The point of using a medicine is to reduce your symptoms, pain, and anxiety to improve your health and quality of life, so if marijuana does not make you feel better it is obviously not the right choice for you.

Chapter 3

What Conditions Can Marijuana Help?

"If marijuana were unknown, and bio-prospectors were suddenly to find it in some remote mountain crevice, its discovery would no doubt be hailed as a medical breakthrough. Scientists would praise its potential for treating everything from pain to cancer, and marvel at its rich pharmacopoeia—many of whose chemicals mimic vital molecules in the human body. In reality, marijuana has been with humanity for thousands of years and is considered by many governments (notably America's) to be a dangerous drug without utility. Any suggestion that the plant might be medically useful is politically controversial, whatever the science says."

—"Reefer Madness: Marijuana Is Medically Useful Whether Politicians Like It or Not," *The Economist* (April 27, 2006)

Wonder Drug?

Can marijuana be the wonder drug to heal your disease and take away all your pain and discomfort? Only occasionally. But for many patients marijuana is an effective medicine that enables them to experience an elevated quality of life. Marijuana has been shown to promote individual healing by making many various symptoms more manageable. When pain and inflammation are effectively managed, the body may begin to heal itself.

Marijuana has been used to treat cancer, control chronic pain, improve mental health, and to address the symptoms of glaucoma, HIV/AIDS, congenital disorders, and gastrointestinal conditions. It may well prove to be a natural and effective therapy for your symptoms.

Marijuana is far safer than most other medicines. Other psychoactive drugs including alcohol, opiates, nicotine, and caffeine have caused fatalities from overdose. According to an FDA report for the years 1990 to 2001, 26,000 people were hospitalized and 458 died each year from overdoses of acetaminophen, the active ingredient in Tylenol. Compare that to the number fatalities from marijuana use—zero. There are zero deaths in recorded history from marijuana overdose. Common substances in our medicine cabinets such as acetaminophen or Vioxx, and recreational intoxicants such as alcohol, are far more dangerous than marijuana and yet are hardly the subject of heated debate. Why then is marijuana so controversial and so misunderstood?

Marijuana Improves Appetite and Decreases Nausea

Eight years ago I was diagnosed with esophageal cancer, a form of cancer with a 95 percent fatality rate. Today I am cancer-free. Initially, I used medical marijuana to counter the nausea from three months of chemotherapy.

Five years ago I had a recurrence and doctors recommended surgery. About 90 percent of my stomach was removed and what was left was reconnected to a shortened esophagus. This was a seven-hour surgery with two surgeons, one working on my stomach and the other opening my back so he could move my lung aside and reconnect my stomach above my diaphragm. When I finally recovered from the surgery, I was left with very little appetite. I can wake up in the morning and not feel hungry until late in the afternoon, and then only a little bit. Medical marijuana gives me the "munchies," so I currently use it to stimulate my appetite.

I have also been left with peripheral neuropathy which makes the top third of my toes constantly tingle. Medical marijuana helps keep my mind off of this condition and focused on my creative work better. It has the same effect on the constant ringing in my ears caused by the chemotherapy.

About six months ago, my oncologist noticed a lighter in my shirt pocket when she was examining me. She asked me if I smoked and I told her about my use of medical marijuana to stimulate my appetite. She told me she would write a prescription for a drug that I could take that would stimulate my appetite instead of the marijuana. She didn't like that I smoked it.

When I looked up the drug on the Internet it turned out to be primarily used as a cancer fighter. It contained progesterone and was designed to make female bodies with breast cancer act like they were pregnant, thereby fighting back the cancer as well as stimulating an appetite. When I told my general practitioner, who had written my recommendation for marijuana, that frankly a couple of tokes usually will do the same thing without my male body being turned into a pregnant female just to stimulate appetite, he said, "Stick with the marijuana."

And I suppose I also use it to help me stay "in the moment" more. As a cancer survivor, my whole life perspective has changed. I truly appreciate the experience of being alive more, and medical marijuana helps me to be more present at any given time. In my daily life, the effects of marijuana provide for a pleasant background to my activities as well as providing a creative jolt to my work as a television and video producer, writer, director, and inventor.

Currently I use a small hash pipe to inhale the smoke. I gave up on rolling and smoking joints when I realized I was burning and inhaling paper along with the marijuana smoke. I can keep a daily supply of medicine in an Altoids tin with the pipe.   —*Ed D, 63*

Symptoms That Marijuana May Relieve

- ADDICTION: Some doctors have reported positive results in curbing patient addiction to various addictive substances including alcohol and opiates. By and large, the drug treatment industry rejects marijuana substitution as a valid treatment for addiction. Unfortunately, there is very little research in this area even though many people have success weaning themselves off other more toxic substances for the less dangerous alternative marijuana.

- ANXIETY, TENSION, AND STRESS: Marijuana has a naturally calming, tranquilizing effect on most people. Some individuals report that it allows them to remain sharper mentally than traditional tranquilizers like Valium, but others report that marijuana creates confusion. These experiences vary individually. Inexperienced or infrequent users of marijuana sometimes experience increased anxiety, self-awareness, or even panic attacks, especially if they use too much too quickly. Some people respond to the unfamiliar feelings by becoming anxious or jittery. As with all psychoactive drugs, a relaxed setting and proper preparation helps avoid these scenarios. More experienced patients find that using marijuana helps them remain calm and relaxed in stressful or anxious situations. Marijuana can reduce tension by helping you to relax your muscles and mind.

- DEPRESSION: Marijuana acts to elevate mood and cope with depression. However, people occasionally experience an increased tendency to become depressed. This is because moods differ widely based on personal outlook, expectations, and the physical environment. Marijuana medicine pioneer and psychiatrist Dr. Tod H. Mikuriya, M.D., (1933-2007) a widely regarded author and advocate for the legalization of marijuana for medical purposes, concluded that marijuana's ability to fight depression is one of its most powerful applications.

◎ DIGESTIVE PROBLEMS: Marijuana is used to treat a number of digestive diseases and conditions. Because of its ability to bind with cannabinoid receptors in the intestines, it relaxes the GI system reducing inflammation, decreasing pain signaling, and increasing nerve-muscle coordination. This results in the digestive system operating more smoothly and regularly. Marijuana renders the symptoms of Crohn's disease and ulcerative colitis much more manageable.

◎ INFLAMMATION: Marijuana's anti-inflammatory properties are unique. Cannabinoids reduce inflammation in joints, which is beneficial to people suffering from arthritis. The way marijuana interacts with the body's receptors and its effects on certain hormones that regulate inflammation make it an outstanding treatment option. Because cannabinoids interact with CB2 receptors in the extremities they can provide localized treatment. Marijuana appears to modulate the body's response to perceived harmful irritants and pathogens. This characteristic can be quite helpful in countering autoimmune conditions such as rheumatoid arthritis and Crohn's disease.

◎ NAUSEA AND VOMITING: Inhaling marijuana works best to treat nausea. For a person experiencing digestive difficulties it is easier to breathe in marijuana vapors than swallow. Inhaling also has a more immediate effect than ingesting a tablet so dosing is easier to control. Inhaling marijuana can help a patient avoid the serious, debilitating effects of vomiting, dehydration, and weight loss.

Another way to administer cannabis for nausea is through the use of sublingual drops. The medicine is absorbed quickly through the mucus membranes, then enters the bloodstream. It never passes through the gastrointestinal tract.

◎ PAIN: Marijuana provides many patients with pain relief. The active ingredients in marijuana work to block the body's pain receptors. Marijuana works best on chronic pain, nerve pain, and pain associated with inflammation. Marijuana is not always as effective as opiates in treating certain pain. However when opiates and cannabinoids are used together the amount of opiates used is reduced substantially.

Marijuana is not addictive or toxic unlike opiates such as morphine and methadone. Combining marijuana and opiates results in greater pain relief as compared to opiates alone. It helps pain sufferers lower their opiate dosage, reducing side-effects. Marijuana works well for the chronic pain of autoimmune diseases such arthritis, swelling, and inflammation, and the severe neuropathic pain that diabetics commonly experience. Marijuana is an effective treatment for migraine headaches.

Marijuana is very effective for pain related to nerve damage and for conditions associated with nerve pain such as MS. It is not as helpful for traumatic or tissue-damaging pains like a broken arm or a severe toothache. However, it is often used for pain associated with old injuries that have not healed correctly, or have developed into arthritis.

⊙ SPASMS AND CONVULSIONS: Conditions that result in muscle spasms or convulsions generally respond positively to marijuana. Patients with these types of disorders are able to reduce or even eliminate the need for toxic prescription medicines. Compared to many prescription drugs, marijuana possesses far more tolerable side effects. Marijuana has been shown to successfully control symptoms related to spasm-inducing disorders such as epilepsy or MS. Ongoing medical studies continue to demonstrate improvements in these symptoms likely via CBD's anticonvulsant properties.

Focusing on the Positives in My Life

I have no other life than my illness. Without the relief of medical marijuana, my life is one long, pain-filled sleepless night plagued with muscle spasms, neck pain, stabbing chest pain, and nightmares.

Due to service-related injuries in the U.S. Navy, I suffer from chronic pain in my back, legs, and chest, which has left me incapable of performing many average everyday functions, which in turn has caused severe depression.

At first, I was prescribed 30mg of morphine twice a day, 550mg of hydrocodone (Vicodin) three times a day. I felt like a junky. I was always sick with cramps and

Conditions Marijuana Benefits

⊙ ARTHRITIS: Arthritis is a devastating disease that makes the patient's world a very uncomfortable and painful place. If you suffer from arthritis, you know that the pain is deep and often unbearable. Most patients suffer from either rheumatoid arthritis or osteoarthritis. Both types impact the joints and cause severe pain, swelling, and limit movement. The pain-relieving qualities of marijuana make it a viable treatment for arthritic pain. Marijuana alone or as an enhancing therapy in conjunction with opioid painkillers can help to manage the pain levels of arthritic conditions. Marijuana's anti-inflammatory properties and ability to regulate some immune system response make it a possible nausea. Eventually my prescription drug use led to three heart attacks.

Marijuana allows me to focus my mind somewhere other then my back pain. Instead of wondering how much relief chewing my right leg off will provide, I can focus on the positive things in my life like my wife and child.

Relief from depression is where marijuana really helps me most. Living in endless pain can make you feel very hopeless. For most of my life I was proud of my body; I was fit and able to stand up straight and tall. Today that isn't the case.

Marijuana provides safer relief from my chronic pain and allows me to be an active participant in my own life once again.   —*Todd, 55*

treatment modality beyond just managing the painful symptoms of arthritis. Marijuana may actually serve to allay the progress of the disease itself. It should be used both internally and in salves to get the medicine to affected areas.

⊚ ATTENTION DEFICIT HYPERACTIVITY DISORDER (ADHD): This disorder of the nervous system is extremely challenging because it makes it difficult to concentrate, complete simple tasks, or clearly focus on assignments. ADHD can manifest in children and carry on into adulthood. Erratic, impulsive behavior and an overactive consciousness can spiral out of control and result in excessive, uncontrollable

Crohn's Disease Symptoms Improved

I was diagnosed with Crohn's disease at the age of 18, less than a week before I moved 300 miles away from my parents' home for college. My first semester was painful and lonely—a complete nightmare.

My immune system was low, and sharing my space with 500 other freshmen meant I was constantly contracting viruses and other contagious illnesses. My large intestine had become covered in scar tissue so thick I couldn't pass food, so I stopped eating.

Eventually, as college continued, I lost 30 pounds and became extremely anemic. During my senior year, when friends on my dorm floor found me passed out in the hallway, I was rushed to the ER. My doctors decided there was no choice left but to remove the section of my

anger or frustration. Marijuana has a calming effect that creates an increased ability to focus on various tasks.

ADHD also affects self-esteem and increases depression. Marijuana is helpful for both conditions. Marijuana is a positive alternative to psychoactive drugs such as Ritalin in treating ADHD.

◉ CANCER TREATMENTS: We have all heard of the nightmarish side effects of chemotherapy and radiation treatments. They are brutal, effectively killing every actively dividing cell in one's body. Marijuana is colon causing the problems. Determined to graduate on time, I scheduled the surgery for spring break, three months away.

I spent those three long months on the steroid prednisone, as well as painkillers and other medications meant to control my symptoms. I gained back the weight immediately, plus some, had violent mood swings, broke out in acne on my face, and had so much water weight in my ankles that when I stood I couldn't walk to class.

After my surgery I saw a doctor and obtained my medical marijuana recommendation. I never needed prednisone again and have not had a serious flare-up in six years. My skin is clear, and my weight is stable.

Today I take Remicade intravenously every eight weeks and supplement the treatment with marijuana tinctures. I've never needed another steroid or painkiller.

—Angelina, 25

an effective treatment to counteract many of the negative side effects of chemo and radiation therapies. Marijuana calms serious nausea, curtails vomiting, and stimulates the appetites of patients experiencing the harsh side effects of these treatments. Both cancer and its treatment are very painful but marijuana eases the suffering. Marijuana treatment also benefits cancer patients who suffer from depression and anxiety as a result of their pain and suffering. Cancer is a life-changing illness and marijuana has been proven to possess the unique ability to make life more tolerable for its sufferers. By alleviating suffering,

Oxycontin and Vicodin vs. Marijuana

When I was 25, my friend and I were in a car accident. He was driving. We clipped another car, spun off the road and flipped. I was ejected from the vehicle and broke every bone below my waist, including my pelvis in nine places. The doctor prescribed a variety of opiate-based medicines, including the infamous Oxycontin and Vicodin. Oxycontin and Vicodin are prescription medications with effects similar to heroin. They are sedatives that corrode the stomach and are extremely addictive. In some areas where I live, Oxycontin is bought and sold widely on the black market and snorted or "free-based."

The side effects of these drugs run the gamut from constipation and stomach ulcers to erectile dysfunction

marijuana allows the patient to focus on the healing instead of the pain and nausea.

⊙ GASTROINTESTINAL DISORDERS: The healing properties of marijuana help to greatly reduce the discomfort of GI disorders. Marijuana works well as a treatment for nausea, vomiting, and pain—all common symptoms associated with gastrointestinal issues. The active ingredients in marijuana treat symptoms common to GI disorders such as Crohn's disease, irritable bowel syndrome, and ulcerative colitis. The cannabinoids bind to receptors in the digestive tract calming spasms, and addiction. The extreme pain coupled with the drugs led to my anxiety and depression. I had smoked marijuana before the accident but stopped for the six months I used the prescription pain medicine. Not only did the medications destroy my body, but they were also extremely expensive and without health insurance, I had to pay for them out of my pocket.

I finally got fed up with spending all of my money on the medications, and a friend offered me some marijuana. It worked. I was able to cut out four of the prescription meds. Even though I still feel pain, marijuana is the only medicine that reduces its intensity but doesn't damage my body. It relieves my anxiety and I am not depressed. If I actually took all the medications they prescribed me, I would be a vegetable. Today, I am motivated to get things done and to live my life.   —*Robert, 28*

mollifying pain, and improving gastric mobility. Marijuana's anti-inflammatory properties make it an ideal treatment option. Marijuana contains immune system modulators that modify immune response, suppressing gastrointestinal discomfort. Marijuana is a popular treatment for GI disorders because it's effective.

⊙ HIV/AIDS: If you or someone you love has been diagnosed with HIV/AIDS, marijuana is a powerful medicine to help overcome the symptoms associated with the disease. Patients often experience a wasting syndrome, wherein their bodies do not process or assimilate nutrition properly. Marijuana stimulates appetite, which makes it easier to eat, and assuages the neuropathic pain associated with the disease. Because of the way it interacts with the cannabinoid receptors in the body, marijuana is extremely effective in regulating the manifestations of this disease.

⊙ INSOMNIA: Not being able to sleep is a widespread problem. It makes you feel powerless, confused, and leaves you exhausted. This fatigue affects all aspects of the sufferer's life. Marijuana helps many people find restful sleep. Whether symptoms from other conditions or just restlessness cause insomnia, marijuana may help you rest better. Some strains of marijuana have a stimulant effect and a strong onset that keeps people awake. For nighttime, a more sedative indica variety is useful. Some patients find that administering marijuana a couple of hours before bed helps them get past the psychoactive properties to the more restful state.

⊙ MIGRAINE: These unbearable and long-lasting headaches are paralyzing and often accompanied by muscle tension and nausea. Many use marijuana to treat these symptoms. Because it can be inhaled or used as a tincture, marijuana works quickly and addresses migraine symptoms almost instantaneously. Marijuana also curbs the debilitating effects of nausea associated with migraines, making it a good choice for this condition. Patients avert the brunt of the migraine headache attack, minimizing both the amplitude of the excruciating pain and the length of its effects by smoking marijuana at the first sign of an attack.

⊙ MOVEMENT DISORDERS: These difficult conditions normally leave patients with impairment or involuntary movements resulting from nerve damage. When these disorders progress simple tasks become extremely difficult. Marijuana is particularly effective in treating spasticity. Movement-related medical conditions impact individuals who have suffered strokes or suffer from multiple sclerosis, cerebral palsy, paraplegia, quadriplegia, and other spinal cord injuries. Most current medical treatments are ineffective in treating spasticity disorders. Cannabinoids possess anti-spasticity, pain-relieving, anti-tremor, and anti-ataxia properties, and relieve debilitating symptoms of movement disorder without the dangerous side effects of prescription medicines.

⊙ MULTIPLE SCLEROSIS: MS is incredibly painful and a difficult disease to manage. This autoimmune disease attacks the central nervous system and, over time, debilitates normal nerve function. Marijuana treats the symptoms by controlling spasticity and relieving tremors in MS patients, as well as treating involuntary muscle contractions that affect speech, eyesight, bladder control, and balance. Marijuana is very effective for the specific type of pain and nerve function disorders associated with MS.

⊙ POST-TRAUMATIC STRESS SYNDROME (PTSS): Traumatic and violent events in your life can leave you debilitated and scarred for long periods of time. Victims of violent crimes or veterans who have seen combat are both likely to suffer from PTSS, also called post-traumatic stress disorder or PTSD. These patients normally suffer from anxiety, depression, sleeplessness, and irritability, and often have difficulty controlling their emotions. Inability to control emotions can leave a PTSS sufferer feeling frustrated, lethargic, and unmotivated. Marijuana maximizes the quality of sleep, as well as suppresses the severity of nightmares, both of which may be helpful in overcoming the symptoms of PTSS. Post-traumatic stress syndrome is often misdiagnosed, so patients are sometimes inappropriately prescribed anti-psychotics and tranquilizers for their symptoms. Marijuana addresses many of the same problems, while allowing a patient to be more active and responsive.

Marijuana Treats
My Multiple Sclerosis

I smoke marijuana to treat my multiple sclerosis. I also use it as a topical ointment to supplement other medications. Having MS is not like having chronic pain. You can seem all right while permanent damage is being done. At any time you can go blind, become paralyzed, and be spastic or weak in one or more body functions. The attacks are very scary, but the idea of silent, accumulating damage is terrifying.

I was diagnosed with MS in 1993. There were no treatments recommended at the time, but I was so concerned that for a year or two I religiously made smoothies with juice, yogurt, and lots of essential fatty acids, based on the idea that fatty acids were necessary for myelin production. With MS, the immune system attacks one's own nervous system causing damage to the fatty covering/insulation on nerves and to the brain's white and grey matter, myelin. I experienced no further symptoms and my doctor told me I had "benign MS," a little known form of MS in which there are no subsequent exacerbations of the disease. I slacked off the EFAs.

Between about 1995 and 1998, I used nothing because I had no symptoms. My second attack in 1998 was frightening, and my doctor recommended I begin treatment with Avonex, an interferon drug. Looking back I realize that early on, it caused spontaneous, intrusive suicidal feelings. I wasn't depressed at the time, so the suicidal feelings with no thoughts or plans of suicide were just plain weird.

The Avonex slowed down the disease progression but didn't entirely stop it. I had other problems with some fatigue and nerve pain and the occasional exacerbation of the disease with noticeable symptoms like weakness. Sometimes these attacks were treated with a rigorous course of intravenous steroids including Solu-Medrol and then prednisone. Steroids have their own nasty side effects: friable veins, psychotic breaks, susceptibility to infections, and more.

Because of problems with the Avonex (a later repeat of the suicidal feelings), I tried Copaxone, but its side effects were not pleasant either. After that I participated in a study for Avonex combined with Tysabri. The Tysabri caused my thyroid to stop working properly, as well as a crippling, can't-get-out-of-bed fatigue and some depression (both probably related to the thyroid problems). Then they prescribed medications to treat my fatigue and depression. What a choice: risk being physically disabled by the MS, or risk the side effects of the MS treatment drugs.

By this time I'd met and observed other people using marijuana and had heard a lot of very convincing testimonials regarding its use for various illnesses. I did my own research on how and why it might work, considered this with what I knew about MS, and weighed the possibilities. I decided to quit the prescription meds—the co-pays were VERY expensive, even with good insurance—and just use marijuana, vitamins, and fatty acids. My results after nine months have been better overall than on the prescription meds, especially when I consider not only the lack of disease progression, but also the lack of side effects, and the much lower cost of treatment.

I do not enjoy the euphoric sensation of recreational marijuana and have experimented with ways to ingest marijuana. I started out using a vaporizer, but today I use a cold-processed glycerite made from the flowers or buds and some leaves. The raw marijuana still has many of the beneficial cannabinoids that work medically without being as psychoactive. I've begun putting more raw marijuana (dried, but I'll use fresh when the time of year allows it) in the blender with juice.

When I switched from prescription medications to marijuana, friends I hadn't seen for awhile all commented on how well I looked. Additionally, I have not felt at all depressed, despite having stopped taking all my prescription medications. It's a subtle, positive effect. You just feel well, and happy, not "drugged." And as I mentioned already, it's a lot less expensive. I love to garden and find it therapeutic, so being able to grow my own feels very holistic and uplifting.

Dr. William Courtney and Kristen Peskuski have been doing research on the cold-pressed glycerite, among other things. Their Marijuana International Web site contains hundreds of research articles, interviews, and lists of resources. http://marijuanainternational.org

—Lacey, 57

Ask a Doctor

As previously stated, marijuana is a relatively safe and natural drug that helps with a number of medical conditions. Because it can cause unwanted side effects in some patients, it is not the best option for everyone. Working closely with a compassionate doctor is the best method for controlling and alleviating your specific symptoms with marijuana.

Operator Error

Marijuana affects everyone differently, but for some it can be an unexpected, profoundly intoxicating, or sedating experience. For others, especially medical users who have chosen a strain specifically to enhance their concentration and relieve pain, it can be a stimulant. Irv Rosenfeld, one of the last four living remaining federal medical marijuana patients, is a good example of this is. Irv does not get high; he smokes marijuana to relieve his pain so he can drive

> Until you know how your chosen medical marijuana affects you, monitor all its effects closely.

more safely. Until you know how your chosen medical marijuana affects you, monitor all its effects closely.

As with any intoxicant, accidents can happen when you are impaired. You have to accept your limitations and identify the effects of particular marijuana strains and dosages on your motor skills and ability to accomplish tasks. Once you have inhaled or ingested medical marijuana do not drive a car, operate heavy machinery, or perform tasks that require a great deal of concentration to insure your and others' safety.

Moderate Dosage with Responsibility

Like any drug, when abused, marijuana can have negative effects on the user. Most of the major issues related to marijuana are minimized with a little common sense. A patient who is educated and aware of marijuana's medical properties generally has a much different experience than a person hoping to party or have a good time. A patient quickly learns how to achieve maximum effect while using as little medicine as possible. Understanding marijuana's effects on your body enables you to know your limitations and plan accordingly.

For many patients, their condition is so severe that marijuana use results in minimal impairment as compared to their symptoms, because it controls their symptoms. For instance, MS patients often find the spasms and pain associated with their illness eliminated. This gives them more control over motor function, making them safer. Each patient should examine both the positive and negative effects of marijuana use on their health and their ability to function when medicated.

Chapter 4

Talking To Your Healthcare Provider and Obtaining Marijuana

Talk to your doctor and find a source for marijuana, but not necessarily in that order. Some people will talk to their doctor before ever bothering to look for marijuana. Others may try marijuana first to see how it works before approaching their doctor. It's like the chicken and the egg—which comes first? It's your choice.

If you decide to try marijuana before seeking professional advice, use it in a familiar setting, in moderation, and with a trusted friend who is not partaking. Never use marijuana in a situation that may endanger yourself or others. If your medical condition is very serious and you don't know how marijuana will interact with your current treatment or impact your health, always consult your physician before experimenting. There are a number of ways to approach your doctor about the subject of using medical marijuana.

Talking To Your Healthcare Provider—Be Prepared

Before discussing medical marijuana with your health care provider, re-

> When you've taken the time to look for reputable sources and provide references, your doctor, nurse practitioner, or physician assistant will take notice because he or she cannot arbitrarily dismiss your concerns.

search the subject thoroughly. Find out if and why marijuana is effective for your particular condition. Be prepared to discuss the information and share the reference for any evidence you discover that proves patients are finding relief using this natural alternative. You can use magazine and medical journal articles, reports, and even personal recommendations to support your position. When you've taken the time to look for reputable sources and provide references, your doctor, nurse practitioner, or physician assistant will take notice because he or she cannot arbitrarily dismiss your concerns. Maybe you'll teach them a thing or two.

Research Sources

The University of California Center for Medicinal Cannabis Research in San Diego keeps an updated list of their International Marijuana Research Society studies online at www.cmcr.ucsd.edu.

Patients Out of Time Web site posts information from its accredited biennial clinical marijuana conference that features leading researchers and clinicians from around the world presenting their new research. The 2006, 2008, and 2010 conference proceedings are available for doctors to watch and earn continuing medical education units. Their conferences are designed for health care professionals. Patients can also view many of the video presentations at www.medicalmarijuana.com.

Doctors Are People Too

Although doctors generally act professionally and are typically thoughtful by nature, they are not immune to the negative stigma associated with marijuana. It is still controversial and your doctor may hold a strong personal bias against it because of his beliefs, experiences, or education. There may be immediate skepticism from your doctor. Don't be alarmed or get discouraged. Allow your doctor to present her or his opinion. If your doctor refuses to have a frank discussion, you have the right as a patient to seek out a second opinion from a physician who is more objective about the value of medical marijuana. Be prepared for disappointment. Many doctors have little real education on the subject. Do you think the doctor's opinion is based on fact and reason or on preconceived prejudices?

Personal Experience

A doctor may dispute a study or attempt to discredit one publication or another, but it's harder to argue against your positive personal experience. It is a powerful statement to say, "I read about it and it seemed just right for my symptoms, so I tried it and it worked." If you try marijuana before consulting your physician, it may be a good idea to keep a written record of your experience—before, during, and after—and especially the medical benefits you notice, and share it with your doctor.

Having this real-life experience to determine whether marijuana helps before discussing it with your doctor eliminates ambiguity about marijuana's efficacy for your condition. Chapter 5 discusses in detail how to use medical marijuana.

Be Smart

If you discuss the option of marijuana with your physician and he or she makes a valid point of why marijuana may not be a good idea for your condition, don't dismiss it just because you want to try it. Your health is at stake so take your trusted physician's opinion into account when making your decision.

Obtaining Marijuana

If you have decided marijuana may help your condition, the next step is to obtain some. Because of its illegal status in some states, accessing it can be a challenge. In some medical marijuana states it is easy to find high quality medicine. If there is no safe access point nearby or you do not live in a state with legal access to marijuana, do not fear. Despite decades of being illegal, high-potency, properly grown, safe marijuana is more readily available than ever. We'll walk you through the legal and unfortunately illegal methods of obtaining medical marijuana.

Legal Methods

Marijuana is a plant, so you can obtain it legally by growing it in states where it is legal to grow for medical use. Some states have passed laws allowing medical marijuana cultivation, use, and distribution, and some have established legal methods of obtaining it as a medicine. Cultivating your own medicine can be challenging and burdensome if you don't have a green thumb or are just not up to it. In medical marijuana states you can access dispensaries, cultivation collectives or cooperatives, delivery services, and caregivers from whom you can obtain medical marijuana legally.

Dispensaries

The most common method of legally providing medical marijuana to patients is through specialty stores called dispensaries. They began in 1994 in California after the founder's partner died of AIDS. At the time marijuana was the only substance that gave HIV/AIDS patients any relief. Dennis Peron's pioneering vision to open a "marijuana club" on Church Street in downtown San Francisco pioneered the model. State drug enforcement agents soon raided this collective in 1996, but its closure resulted in a proliferation of medical marijuana services that continue to impact medical treatment worldwide. Thousands of dispensaries provide medicine in California, Colorado, Michigan, Nevada, Oregon, Washington, and other states, and in many other countries.

Dispensaries provide a wide variety of medical marijuana products including marijuana buds, which are usually smoked or vaporized (see Chapter 5), concentrates of the buds such as hashish, kief, oil extractions, tinctures, drinks, and edibles, and topical salves to patients. These outlets operate much like ordinary retail pharmacies. Depending on the state they require a doctor's or a healthcare professional's recommendation rather than a prescription. Once you have the documentation the dispensary can provide you medical marijuana products.

There are many different dispensary models but their common goal is to provide marijuana to patients in need. Some have adopted a total wellness treatment approach complete with massage therapy, support group meetings, and counseling. Others have more express service that allows patients to access their medicine quickly and often at lesser expense because of their lower overhead. A number of interesting and unique dispensary models are evolving. If you are fortunate enough to live in an area with multiple dispensaries, visit several to find the one that best suits you.

One major difference between a dispensary and a traditional pharmacy is the services they provide. Your recommendation will not specify the type of marijuana to use as they would prescribe a specific pain medicine. The healthcare professional can only recommend that you use medical marijuana for your condition, but not the strain. An educated, experienced dispensary staff can help guide you when choosing specific medicines that will help you. Finding a dispensary with a friendly, knowledgeable staff can help you achieve optimum success with medical marijuana.

When you enter a dispensary for the first time, you may be a bit overwhelmed. Maybe you've never purchased marijuana before, or perhaps you've never seen so many options in one place. The benefit of a good, well-stocked dispensary is that it can provide lots of variety so patients can receive customized treatment. A traditional marijuana dealer may have one or two strains, whereas a good dispensary has 20 to 30 strains available. Even though different marijuana strains have some common traits, patients often find more therapeutic value for their condition in one strain rather than another. If you find that certain marijuana strains are more effective for treating your particular condition, the dispensary will try to provide a consistent supply of that specific medicine for you. The development of new targeted strains provides patients with faster, more effective, medical results.

Most dispensaries carry whole raw plant medicines including marijuana flowers or buds as well as a variety of products containing marijuana. Local regulations and guidelines vary, so product selection varies. Select a dispensary that offers a wide selection of medicines such as extractions, tinctures or topical ointments, and ingestibles. Chapter 6 covers these different types of marijuana medication.

To find out what the laws are in your area regarding dispensaries, visit www.AmericansForSafeAccess.org. There are also many good Internet sites such as www.weedmaps.com and www.stickyguide.com that list medical marijuana dispensaries.

Cultivation Collectives or Cooperatives

In some states dispensaries are also growing collectives or cooperatives. These are non-retail groups of patients and providers who share resources and the bounty of collective gardens. A good example is the Wo/Men's Alliance for Medical Marijuana (WAMM) in Santa Cruz, California. It is the nation's oldest medical marijuana collective that serves patients directly. Their model is based on their belief that all patients cannot grow marijuana, either because of medical conditions or lack of time, skills, or resources. Those members who can't grow can provide other resources like money, space, equipment, or supplies. Those with more skill or energy can cultivate and harvest the plants for use by the entire collective. WAMM periodically holds meetings to distribute the medicine to its patient members and in some cases they provide critical end-of-life care for people and distribute the medicine to them.

Cultivation collectives or co-ops may consist of a few patients who join forces to produce for and provide medicine to one another or they can include several hundred patients who share resources. Many charge "incremental reimbursement" fees to members to ensure fairness, allowing patients who use more medicine to give more financial support to the effort.

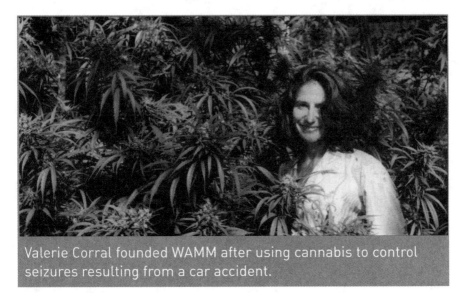

Valerie Corral founded WAMM after using cannabis to control seizures resulting from a car accident.

Other members are responsible for doing the work and are compensated for their efforts. Cultivation collectives or cooperatives provide a more personal relationship between the patient and the people who grow the medicine. Members sometimes make the finished foods or other oils, butters, or tinctures sold through the co-op. On the other hand, there are often fewer marijuana varieties available than offered by a dispensary. People in a co-operative usually know each other through their social network. Compared to public organizations or retail stores, these organizations are intimate and private with regular meetings and member voting rights.

Delivery Services

The delivery service model is emerging as a popular method for people to access medical marijuana. Often referred to as "in-home care services," these organizations cater to individual members who prefer their medicine be delivered directly to their home. Some members may lack mobility; others desire to keep their medical need for marijuana private. Some patients are not comfortable going to a store or a meeting where they may run into people from their community. Many delivery services also offer a wide selection of medical marijuana and finished medicated products. You can find the delivery services listed on the same Web sites and printed lists where dispensary locations are available, such as www.weedmaps.com.

Caregivers

State and local governments require varying levels of services that must be provided to the patient in order to be considered a "caregiver." In some states, one needs only to provide medical marijuana to a patient, whereas in other states one may be required to consistently assume the housing, health, or security responsibility for the patient's care. Regardless of the local legal definition, the caregiver's role is to obtain and administer marijuana to the patient because of the patient's medical condition or because the patient is incapable of growing the marijuana plants. Patients with mobility issues can assign a caregiver to go to a dispensary or other outlets and make decisions on their behalf.

Depending on state definition, a caregiver relationship may be a one-on-one relationship between the patient and an individual who aids them in everyday life. In some states caregivers may care for many patients and in others there may be more defined restrictions. Many patients cultivate or obtain medicine for other patients in the caregiver system. These relationships may be formed with people the patient already knows who cultivate medical marijuana, with a person referred by a friend, or through the patient and caregiver's mutual social network. Finding someone you trust to obtain or grow quality medicine for you is a good option if you desire a more personal relationship with the person who produces or acquires your medical marijuana supply.

Even though we use the term "legally," marijuana is still very much illegal under federal law. Patients must never put themselves in harm's way to provide or receive medicine. Federal drug agents usually focus on larger cases, not medical marijuana patient possession, but there is always the threat of federal law enforcement.

Illegally

Unfortunately, in non-medical marijuana states, obtaining medicine from unlawful sources is a major problem routinely faced by many patients. There is no easy or safe access to a wide range of varieties of marijuana and marijuana medicines. Even in some states with medical marijuana laws, systems are not in place to provide safe marijuana access to patients. This forces many patients to depend on illegal resources to obtain medicine.

In spite of the war on drugs, there is plenty of marijuana available on the black market. Chances are, you know someone who knows someone who can get marijuana for you to use as a medicine. Perhaps you know that someone yourself. Most people who sell marijuana are otherwise law-abiding citizens trying to pay for their own marijuana by purchasing in bulk and selling to others in smaller increments. Even with good contacts there are still inherent dangers to acquiring medicine on the black market.

> Unfortunately, in non-medical marijuana states, obtaining medicine from unlawful sources is a major problem routinely faced by many patients.

Ask Around

Most likely, there is someone in your immediate group of friends who has access to marijuana and you likely have a hunch they've used it themselves. Younger people are more likely to know where to find marijuana because it is culturally acceptable. It is not wise to ask people you do not know well about buying marijuana. It could make them feel uncomfortable, or even get you in significant trouble with the law.

Be Safe

Never venture into dangerous areas or involve yourself with nefarious characters to obtain marijuana. Although maintaining your health is paramount, there are many untrustworthy hucksters and charlatans out there. Be sure to search for a reputable source for your medicinal marijuana. Take pains to find a safe, honest person who understands your medical need. Use your gut instincts to make wise choices to obtain your medicine.

Buying in Bulk

Like most products, you can get a better deal if you buy marijuana in bulk. When you are buying marijuana from an illegal source you may be limited by the amount available. From a legal standpoint, most law enforcement considers buying one ounce, 28.5 grams, or less to be a minor crime. Buying an ounce, instead of 28 separate grams, you gain considerable savings.

Growing Illegally

Sometimes the safest, most reliable way of obtaining marijuana is to grow it yourself, especially if you live in an area that does not have medical marijuana laws. However, cultivators are subject to serious penalties in some states. Be aware of the possible consequences and weigh those against your medical necessity. Discussing your desire to grow illegally with the people closest to you is a good idea because they too will suffer if you are prosecuted. Take your loved one's advice; they want to end your suffering as much as you. Weigh the risk to your livelihood, freedom, or standing within your family or community

Your Safety First

Whether you're gardening indoors or out, your safety is of the utmost concern. There are many devices that mask or remove the smell of marijuana to avoid detection, such as charcoal filters, negative ion generators, and anti-scent gels. Never tell people about your garden. Many marijuana cultivators are arrested because they told someone who told someone else. Loose lips may also result in break-ins at your grow site. People steal marijuana because of its high value on the black market. Take all possible precautions to keep your garden protected from detection by law enforcement, shady acquaintances, neighbors, and burglars.

How Was the Medical Marijuana Grown and Handled?

The above list of methods of obtaining medical marijuana has relevance beyond the legal ramifications—how your marijuana was grown and handled during harvest and shipment can affect your health. Where marijuana is illegal, the cultivation and production is rarely regulated. When marijuana is purchased on the black market instead of grown and distributed legally, the potential for chemical or biological contamination is present. Unethical practices may never be discovered because there is no random or required testing of these products in the supply line before they get to the patient. Fortunately, contamination problems are not common.

In states where marijuana is legal for medical use, quality control methods and product testing assure a safer supply of medical marijuana. In some areas of California, dispensaries and cooperatives are required to have medicine screened for toxins and contaminants by a third-party laboratory. These tests protect patients from marijuana contaminated with mold and mildew from poor growing conditions or improper curing. Further, some growers may use

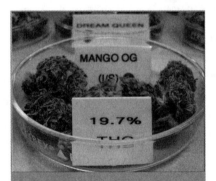

This THC level of this strain of Mango tests at 19.7%. A high THC percentage means that less may be needed for therapeutic results.

PHOTO: RACHAEL SZMAJDA

chemicals to combat pests or powdery mildew. This could surely compromise the health of an already sick patient. The labs also screen for potency, providing patients with information that helps them manage their dosage.

If your locale has dispensaries, ask a representative at your local dispensary if they use a laboratory service or have one on the premises. Many established dispensaries now use laboratory testing to determine if marijuana has been treated with pesticides or other chemicals that are unsafe. These dispensaries do not carry unsafe medicine for their patients and are a better choice over dispensaries that do not test medicine for resale.

TESTING

In California and Colorado, patients using medical marijuana have the added security of laboratory-tested marijuana. Not only does the testing lab certify a hygienic product, but it also measures the levels of THC, CBD, and CBN in the medicine, which provides patients with more information.

In places with a legal market, lab testing has become industry standard, pushing growers to produce clean and healthful medicine.

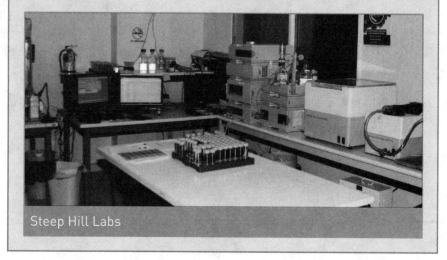

Steep Hill Labs

Chapter 5

How to Use Medical Marijuana

After weighing the pros and cons and discussing it with your physician, you've decided medical marijuana may benefit you. You've located a trustworthy source, you've procured your medicine, and now you're ready to try it for the first time.

Finding the right type, the right dosage, and the right method for using medical marijuana are imperative to achieving the greatest relief possible. Understanding the most appropriate method of intake for your particular condition is important to achieve the most therapeutic use from marijuana. Most people are familiar with smoking marijuana; however, eating marijuana in food or using it as a topical treatment has specific, targeted benefits for particular symptoms and conditions.

Keep in mind every person has a different body chemistry and metabolism, which shapes an individual's reaction to marijuana. What works for someone else may not be the best option for you. If you try administering marijuana one way and don't achieve the effects you desire, it's possible another delivery method may be a better option. Don't get discouraged. Just as with any pharmaceutical regimen it may take time to dial in the most efficacious way to use marijuana for your specific symptoms.

Inhalation

Inhaling marijuana provides nearly instant relief. The effects of inhaling marijuana smoke or vapor are virtually immediate, so in case of nausea or rapid-onset migraine symptoms, the active ingredients can be administered into your system before your symptoms become too profound. Patients report avoiding a more traumatic experience by taking one or two puffs of marijuana smoke or vapor as soon as they begin to notice symptoms. These first crucial moments might prove the difference between a mild attack and a severe one.

For cancer patients undergoing chemotherapy and radiation treatments, the ability to inhale medicine that works immediately to stop nausea before it turns into full-blown vomiting is an amazing alternative to pill-based medications. Patients can retain the nourishment from food and avoid the violent, debilitating convulsions associated with protracted vomiting. The inability to keep down food can result in severe weight loss and wasting in some patients, which can badly compromise their body's natural ability to heal itself. Patients who suffer from nausea and vomiting cringe at the idea of swallowing anything, so inhaling medicine is an optimal delivery method. The two most common methods of inhalation are smoking and vaporizing.

> The two most common methods of inhalation are smoking and vaporizing.

Smoking Marijuana

Smoking marijuana is by far the most common delivery method because it's easy and inexpensive. However, smoking may be uncomfortable for non-experienced people.

What about the comparison of tobacco smoke and marijuana smoke? Are parallels as to the dangers of the intake levels of carcinogens and tar

LARGE STUDY FINDS NO LINK
BETWEEN MARIJUANA AND LUNG CANCER

The smoke from burning marijuana leaves contains several known carcinogens and the tar it creates contains 50 percent more of some of the chemicals linked to lung cancer than tobacco smoke. A marijuana cigarette also deposits four times as much of that tar as an equivalent tobacco cigarette. Scientists were therefore surprised to learn that a study of more than 2,000 people found no increase in the risk of developing lung cancer for marijuana smokers.

"We expected that we would find that a history of heavy marijuana use—more than 500 to 1,000 uses—would increase the risk of cancer from several years to decades after exposure to marijuana," explains lung researcher Dr. Donald Tashkin of the University of California, Los Angeles, and lead researcher on the project. But looking at residents of Los Angeles County, the scientists found that even those who smoked more than 20,000 joints in their lifetimes did not have an increased risk of lung cancer.

The researchers interviewed 611 lung cancer patients and 1,040 healthy controls as well as 601 patients with cancer in the head or neck region under the age of 60 to create the statistical analysis. They found that 80 percent of those with lung cancer and 70 percent of those with other cancers had smoked tobacco, although only roughly half of both groups had smoked marijuana.

But after controlling for tobacco, alcohol, and other drug use, as well as matching patients and controls by age, gender, and neighborhood, marijuana did not seem to have an effect, despite its unhealthy aspects. "Marijuana is packed more loosely than tobacco, so there's less filtration through the rod of the cigarette, so more particles will be inhaled," Tashkin says. "And marijuana smokers typically smoke differently than tobacco smokers. They hold their breath about four times longer allowing more time for extra fine particles to deposit in the lungs."

Tashkin speculates that perhaps the THC chemical in marijuana smoke prompts aging cells to die before becoming cancerous. Tashkin and his colleagues presented the findings yesterday at a meeting of the American Thoracic Society in San Diego.

—David Biello, *Scientific American* (May 24, 2006)

valid? Consider this. Because it takes very little marijuana smoke to achieve the desired results, the volume of marijuana smoke inhaled, as compared to tobacco smoke, is dramatically lower. A cigarette smoker can easily inhale an ounce or more of tobacco per day, but it is rare that a marijuana smoker will inhale an ounce of marijuana per *week*. It's just not necessary to smoke that much marijuana. The availability of more potent marijuana strains during recent years means you don't need to take in as much smoke to get the desired medicinal results. Just to make the point, a chronic cigarette smoker might take in one or two packs of cigarettes daily each at 20 cigarettes per pack and approximately 10 lungfuls per cigarette, the equivalent to 200 to 400 lungfuls of smoke per day. In stark comparison, a medicinal marijuana user might only require one or two lungfuls of marijuana smoke to feel the full effects of their medicine, the effects of which may last many hours or even all day. Considering there is no trace of the carcinogen nicotine in marijuana smoke, it seems that smoking marijuana is nowhere near as dangerous as smoking tobacco.

Methods of Ingestion

Generally medical marijuana is smoked in a cigarette, a pipe, or a water-filtrated pipe or device. There are many creative methods by which people can smoke marijuana but we'll stick to the basics.

- ◉ MARIJUANA CIGARETTES OR CIGARS: Wrapping marijuana into a cigarette paper is the most common method of smoking because it's cheap, simple, effective, and easy to dispose of or conceal. A pack of cigarette rolling papers doesn't cost much but rolling a good cigarette takes practice. Break up the marijuana and wrap a rolling paper around it. Compared to a pipe, the cigarette, or joint, may use more marijuana because it continues to burn between inhalations.

- ◉ PIPES AND SUCH: Regardless of its form, it's easier to control the amount of smoke you take in using a pipe. Your pipe can be a very small "one-hitter" or an elaborate glass piece. Even a traditional corn-cob pipe will do. Smoking medical marijuana from a glass pipe is more common because of the clean taste. Also, it's safer because the glass doesn't react or burn in the presence of extreme heat.

⊚ WATER FILTRATION PIPES: These smoking devices are known as "waterpipes," "bongs," and "bubblers." A bong is a larger device than a bubbler and has a bowl on a hollow stem that goes down into a chamber area where water is stored. Upon lighting marijuana in the bowl area and inhaling, suction pulls the smoke through the water and into your lungs, thus filtering out most of the particulates in the smokestream and cooling it. Some people add ice to their bong apparatus for a smoother, even cooler, smoke. Bongs come in all shapes and sizes, from utilitarian columns to expansive glass creations to any number of ce-ramic art pieces with a bowl in one area and a mouthpiece in the other. Some bongs have remov-able "down-stems," or bowls that enable airflow to clear the smoke from the chamber. Others have carburetor holes that are cov-ered with one finger while draw-ing smoke into the chamber and then released to clear the smoke-filled chamber. Some bongs are downright complex. A bubbler is a simple, smaller, pipe-sized, wa-ter-filtered smoking device, usu-ally glass with a smaller chamber area; bubblers are also carburet-ed to clear the chamber.

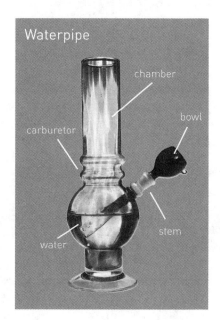

Waterpipe

chamber

bowl

carburetor

stem

water

Choosing a smoking implement is your choice, although anything at your local shop will likely do the trick. A $2 pipe will administer your medicine as well as a $2,000 custom-made bong. Smoking marijuana has some risk. Inhaling the pyrolyzed fumes of any burning organic matter is suboptimal. There are safer options such as vaporization or ingestion, which may be just as effective as smoking without the potential for lung irritation.

HOW TO USE A PIPE

Put the marijuana into the bowl of the pipe. The bowl is connected to a mouthpiece where you place your lips to draw in the air and smoke. With a lighter or a match ignite the marijuana and gently breathe in. When you feel you have inhaled enough, cover the bowl area, reducing the oxygen supply to extinguish the smoldering marijuana, a technique that enables you to use less medical marijuana per smoking session. Using this method you can easily monitor your intake and add smaller or larger amounts to the bowl to meet your optimal medical needs. Pipes are versatile, user-friendly, and efficient. You can find marijuana pipes at most smoke shops in most cities. Some states and towns have restrictive drug paraphernalia laws that limit your selection.

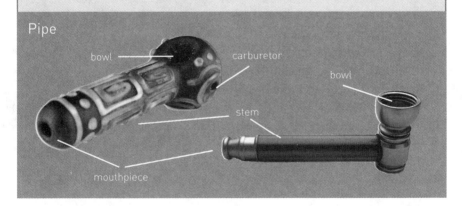

Pipe

bowl

carburetor

bowl

stem

mouthpiece

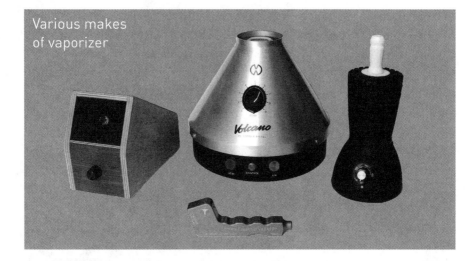

Various makes of vaporizer

Vaporizing Marijuana

A vaporizer is a device that heats marijuana to a temperature that turns the THC and other cannabinoids into vapor without burning because vaporization takes place at a lower temperature than a burn. Vaporizers can significantly reduce the intake of the harsh compounds associated with burning organic material and still provide the rapid onset and easy dose management associated with marijuana inhalation. The drawback is that vaporization requires equipment.

An array of choices is available including portable devices that provide adequate medication delivery discreetly and larger tabletop units better suited for home use. There also are more technologically advanced fixture devices that regulate the temperature more precisely. All vaporizers do the same thing: They heat the plant material to a temperature that evaporates or boils the liquid oils, creating a vapor containing terpenes and cannabinoids but no pyroletic products. It is a lighter effect, which is summarily different from smoking and can take some getting used to if you are accustomed to smoking. It's like water flavored with essences as compared with a soda.

The health benefits of this method are obvious and patients have even been allowed to use vaporizers in hospitals. Some devices are direct heat-to-inhalation devices; others capture the vapor in a bag or balloon of some sort and allow the patient to regulate intake. Vaporizers continue to evolve as the preferred and most recommended medical delivery method because of their comparative safety and ability to deliver a rapid response.

Extractions

Extractions, also called concentrates or tinctures, are derived from the marijuana plant but do not contain actual plant material. Extractions contain only the active ingredients, leaving the plant behind. The medical benefits are clear: Patients who need a stronger dosage can consume it without also consuming plant matter. Common methods of extraction are cold water extraction, evaporative extraction, dry tumbling (or "kiefing"), and direct contact extraction. The end products created using these methods are liquids, oils, resins, and powdery compositions commonly referred to as hashish (hash), kief, honey oil, or hash oil.

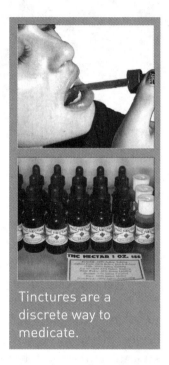

Tinctures are a discrete way to medicate.

Extracts can be smoked, eaten in foods, or applied topically. Some aren't recommended for use in foods because potentially dangerous solvents are used in their production. Others do not vaporize well because of their high moisture content. Here are some methods used to create different marijuana extractions.

⊚ COLD WATER EXTRACTION HASH: The process of making water hash is relatively simple and produces an excellent product. A series of nylon bags with different size screens on the bottom are used to catch different size particulates. Plant materials such as trimmings and small buds are placed into the bags with ice and water. The mixture is agitated and then strained through the bag with the largest screen size. The residue-filled cold water is strained though the next size bag and then the next, leaving a different quality of residue in each bag. The last couple bags usually contain the highest concentration of active ingredients and the least amount of waxes, plant residues, and chlorophyll. Then the end product from each bag is dried and rolled into a solid piece. It can be smoked, eaten, or used in other applications. If the hash still contains much moisture, vaporizing it can be difficult.

One advantage of the water process is that the water washes the glands so fungal spores and other contaminants are rinsed away. This results in a very pure uncontaminated product. It can be smoked or ingested in food.

◉ KIEF OR DRY SIFT RESIN: The word kief refers to either the resin glands of the mature female marijuana plant or a powder made from those glands. Kief is prized for its smooth smoke. To make the dry, fluffy kief powder, the glands are separated from the plant material—usually "trash" buds and leaves—using a screen or a screen-lined tumbler. The golden dust contains a higher level of concentrated cannabinoids than the bud material. Kief is versatile and can be administered in a number of methods. Because it is so dry, it can result in a harsher smoke, and because no solvent is used in the extraction process, it is safe to use in food.

◉ HASH OIL: Hash oil is commonly made by combining marijuana and alcohol and heating it over low heat for a long period of time to evaporate the solvent. After the plant material is removed what is left is an oily residue high in THC and other active ingredients. The oil can be smoked or vaporized. It's best to use grain alcohol, which is the alcohol humans consume, as the solvent. Cheaper, poisonous isopropyl alcohol is sometimes used, and is dangerous to ingest, so you must be sure all the solvent is evaporated. Hash oil is usually smoked or vaporized and sometimes used by commercial kitchens in preparing edibles.

⊙ TINCTURES: Tinctures are made by concentrating the cannabinoids dissolved in the alcohol-cannabis extraction. Sometimes the alcohol is replaced with vegetable glycerin. The advantage of a tincture is that it isn't ingested and has a fast action time, second only to inhalation. The feeling it creates is similar to smoking a joint rather than the slightly different feeling produced through ingesting.

⊙ CONTACT HASH: The simplest hashing technique known, making contact hash involves rubbing plant material with the hands or an instrument to remove the resinous trichomes. In some parts of the world people rub the marijuana plant with their hands or with leather and then roll the residue into sticky balls. This substance is pure resin from the plant so it is especially safe.

Food-Based Medicines

When you think of eating marijuana, the iconic pot brownie probably comes to mind. However, marijuana extracts can be infused into common cooking ingredients such as butter and oils and then used to cook into any food or added to beverages. Medical marijuana foods are often referred to collectively as "edibles." Cannabinoids are fatty by nature, and bond easily to the fats in butter, oil, and creams, or to glucose.

To ingest marijuana, you can't just dump it raw into food and eat it because

Eating marijuana has a much longer onset when compared to the effects of inhaling smoke or vapor.

it's bitter, fibrous, and difficult to digest. Removing the active cannabinoids and including them in recipes results in tasty foods. Butter is the most common ingredient used to extract cannabinoids because of tradition and its high fat content, but vegetable oils such as olive oil are more effective.

Usually dried leaves, rather than buds, are used because they are much less expensive and cost less per gram of cannabinoids than the buds. Remove all stems and seeds. Some people grind it up using a blender, other cooks leave the leaves whole or just chop them into small pieces. Heat the butter or oil mix after weighing the material so you will be able to determine portion size later. The oil or butter and ground leaf mixture will barely simmer for about an hour. Then filter the plant matter from the marijuana-infused butter or oil. This infused fat can then be added to your favorite food recipe for a delightful way to take your medicine.

It is important to monitor the dosage in marijuana-laden foods. By measuring the amount of marijuana and butter or oil used to make the solution you can figure the number of grams of marijuana used for each measure. For instance, if you used an ounce of marijuana and 10 ounces of oil, each ounce would contain the THC from 2.8 grams of marijuana, which is a moderate portion for a person who weighs about 150 pounds. An average amount of intake is about a gram for every 50 pounds of weight.

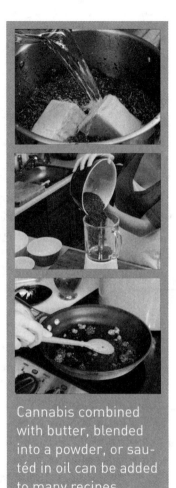

Cannabis combined with butter, blended into a powder, or sautéd in oil can be added to many recipes.

PHOTO: JOE BURULL

RATIO CHART FOR INCREASING OR DECREASING POTENCY

STRENGTH	BUDS/FLOWERS	LEAF TRIM/SHAKE
Maximum Strength Formula	1 Ounce	4 Ounces
High Strength Formula	¾ Ounce	3 Ounces
Elevated Strength Formula	½ Ounce	2 Ounces
Low Strength Formula	¼ Ounce	1 Ounce

The safest way to experiment with edible marijuana is through self-titration: that is, by partaking of small amounts first. Begin by sampling a very small portion and then wait an hour for the medicine to take full effect. Eating marijuana has a much longer onset when compared to the effects of inhaling smoke or vapor. It is easy to take in too much while anticipating the onset of the effects. Give yourself an hour to feel the full effect, longer if you have a gastrointestinal malady that slows down your digestive processes.

After you feel the full effect of your edibles, you can then make a decision on whether to use more or less next time.

The feeling from eating marijuana is qualitatively different than inhaling or using a tincture. The THC is converted in the intestines to a metabolite commonly called 11-Hydroxyl(THC) and written 11-0H-THC.

Eating marijuana has a much deeper effect, affecting the body more than inhalation. It can be temporarily immobilizing if too much is used. A large dose of ingested marijuana can result in a mild hallucinogenic effect, a feeling many find disconcerting. However, eating marijuana is safer than inhaling and the medicinal effects last as much as twice as long. *If you have eaten too much, there is no harm done. You will probably feel dreamy or tired. Go with the flow and relax. The feeling will wear off within a few hours and your body will have no ill effects from the experience. Unless there are symptoms such as tremors (the result of an extremely high overdose) or other threatening physical symptoms, there is no need to seek medical treatment. The unusual feelings will abate naturally.*

Finding the appropriate edible dosage

I had never smoked marijuana before and was not keen on the idea of smoking anything; I had never even smoked a cigarette.

After suffering from arthritis for about a year I decided to try marijuana. A friend had introduced me to vaporizing, which did in fact provide relief. I was able to pick up a pen or pencil and write birthday and holiday cards for my grandchildren without pain.

Although vaporizing worked I was more interested in ingesting marijuana in food rather than going to the trouble of purchasing and operating a vaporizer. The first time I made my own "edibles," I made them entirely too strong, which was incredibly uncomfortable. I now know the appropriate level of dosage for me. I make a batch of cookies once a month and have not had another bad experience with marijuana.

—Edna, 76

Treating Symptoms of Psoriasis

I use medical marijuana to treat the symptoms of psoriasis. Psoriasis is a genetic autoimmune condition that causes skin redness, irritation, and flaky silver patches called "scale." Although common, it has no cure and flare-ups can be triggered by anything from stress to medications, alcohol or even too much sun. Besides being uncomfortable and irritated from dry, flaky skin, sometimes I feel shunned like a leper. Most people assume it's contagious.

I smoke marijuana to treat the stress and anxiety that cause flare-ups. Doctors typically prescribe steroid creams or pharmaceuticals to manage the symptoms. However, I have found that using topical treatments derived from marijuana are the most effective way to treat my symptoms. For the most part, I am able to keep my psoriasis at bay and avoid major flare-ups.

I also like to make my own topical ointments. The marijuana can be extracted for a natural topical treatment. I grind up the buds or leaf and infuse it with olive oil. After three to four hours in a slow cooker, I strain out the leaf and herbal material. I mix the cooled product with raw shea butter or apply it directly to the skin. Sometimes for added relief or aromatherapy I add essential oils of lavender or spearmint. It provides instant relief and smells great as well!

—Annabelle, 27

Topical Applications

Marijuana can be used in oils, salves, and compounds that are applied directly to the skin. Many patients report that these medicines act to reduce aches and pains, improve dryness in skin, and help treat sores and disorders. Topical applications have no known psychoactive effects but have proven effective in addressing a variety of skin and muscle symptoms.

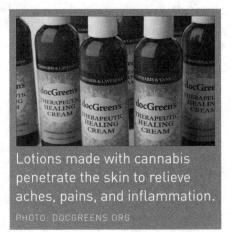

Lotions made with cannabis penetrate the skin to relieve aches, pains, and inflammation.

PHOTO: DOCGREENS.ORG

Safe Use Principles

The most important part of using marijuana, no matter how you choose to take it, is to maintain a safe environment to ensure a satisfying experience. Medicine is supposed to be helpful; it makes sense that using marijuana medicinally is not the same as using it recreationally. Many medical patients benefit from the medicinal properties of the marijuana plant. The euphoria created is not the same as with a non-patient, much like the pain-alleviating experience of prescription opiates for the chronic pain sufferer is categorically different from the experience of a morphine addict getting their fix. But like so many other psychoactive medicines, there is potential for abuse of cannabinoid medications. For some it might be difficult to distinguish between reasonable medical dosages and recreational usage.

Always use marijuana in a safe familiar setting to be sure your experience is positive. Do not partake of a dissociating dose of marijuana and then attempt a complex, potentially dangerous activity such as driving a motor vehicle. Avoid places where your presence might create a disturbance or attract the attention of law enforcement. Learn to utilize your medicine properly and within the accepted norms of your environment.

Chapter 6

Marijuana the Plant and Its Varieties

To the naked eye, the marijuana plant appears to be just a classic plant with the usual leaves, stems, roots, and flowers. However, its chemical property—the production of cannabinoids—is unique in the plant world. In this chapter we'll examine its structure, growth, reproduction, and the classification of marijuana. Not all marijuana is created equal so we'll examine some of the varieties that produce diverse therapeutic effects.

The Plant

Marijuana is a flowering annual so it germinates, grows, flowers, and dies in one season. Unlike other annuals it is dioecious; each individual plant is distinctly male or female, like mammals. It cannot self-pollinate. The males' pollen is spread by the wind. After pollination the females produce seeds. Marijuana can be grown from a seed or a cutting. When a seed is planted, it germinates. The seedling displays the plant model: stem and leaves above ground and a root system below. The leaves gather the light used by the plant for photosynthesis, a process in which the plant uses primarily red and blue light to combine carbon dioxide gas and water into sugar, which is used for both energy and growth. Seedlings grow rapidly with the right conditions. Branches grow from the stem. Characteristically marijuana leaves have five to seven serrated blades with fine sawtooth-like edges. The leaves become larger and are either narrower or wider depending on variety. The plant grows into a bush-like structure and the female plants produce a stunning, pungent flower.

> Not all marijuana is created equal.

Marijuana goes through separate vegetative and flowering stages. During the vegetative stage the plant uses all of its energy to grow as large as possible. Then it transitions into the flowering phase. It redirects its energy into producing flowering clusters of buds along the nodes.

When grown naturally outdoors, the vegetative growth phase occurs in spring or early summer. Then the plants flower. They ripen and are harvested in the fall, at the end of the flowering phase. Marijuana is a short-day plant; it measures the length of the uninterrupted dark period, or night, to determine when it's time to reproduce. Longer nights and shorter days signal the plant to begin to flower so seeds will be produced before the onset of winter.

Both indoors and out, the light cycle can be manipulated to force the plants to move from the vegetative to the flowering stage. The flowers develop in small bunches. These tuft-like formations produce colorful, aromatic buds with unique traits that define different plant strains. The female plant produces the desired resinous flowers ideal for medical use. If a male plant does not pollinate the female plant, the resulting unpollinated flowers will be seedless. Seeded buds are undesirable because the smoke generated by burning seeds is acrid, hot, and has no medical usefulness. Redirecting a female plant's energy into creating cannabinoid-rich buds rather than generating seeds for reproduction makes for more viable, medically useful marijuana. It also results in vastly increased yields of useable material. These buds are called sinsemilla, Spanish for "without seeds." However, seeded marijuana is still just fine as medicine if you simply remove the seeds before use. Seeds are useful for breeders and some cultivators.

Marijuana plants vary in size and stature depending on genetic makeup and growing conditions. Some varieties grow tall and lanky and others grow short and thick. Outdoors a marijuana plant grows between 4 to 12 feet tall in a full growing cycle. Some giants have been bred to reach 20 foot height with diameters as large as 10 feet. An indoor garden plant is typically trained and trimmed down to be smaller, between 2 to 6 feet because the vegetative cycle is shorter to allow for more frequent harvests. Marijuana grows vigorously to fit the growing space. Outdoors the stem of a giant can grow to a diameter of 5 inches. It is extremely strong—hence its historical use as a fiber source. Marijuana plants can survive in many conditions.

Taxonomy

Taxonomy is the classification system biologists use to name organisms in order to define differences and show relationships.

Kingdom-	Plantae	Plants
Subkingdom	Tracheobionta	Vascular plants have a system to circulate liquids
Division	Magnoliophyta	Flowering plants
Class	Magnoliopsida	Dicots—pairs of leaves
Order	Rosales	Has certain internal nitrogen fixing
Family	Cannabaceae	Palmate leaves, stipules (hairs and tri-chomes). Includes hops, hackberries
Genus	Cannabis L.	Includes all varieties of marijuana and hemp
Species	Cannabis sativa L	Includes all varieties of marijuana and hemp
Subspecies	Indica, Sativa, Ruderalis	Results of human intervention

Sativa

Sativa plants are taller than either indica or ruderalis. They are thinner with more space between branches, which makes them seem less full. Some sativa strains grow tall, wide, and spindly. Their leaves have fingers that are long and thin with serrated edges. The plant bears large, long, thin flower clusters known as colas.

Sativa-dominant strains have a light, heady feeling. It's an effect that feels more brain- than body-dominant. Sativas provide a more uplifting experience than indica varieties. The sativa effect is more desirable for daytime or active hours because it doesn't affect your ability to work or function. Still, it provides potent pain relief. This heady effect may be a contraindication for some patients since it can cause them feelings of anxiety. They require a calming or relaxing strain.

People experience sativa varieties as daydreamy, intellectual, and inquisitive. They can be flighty to intense. Pure sativas are hard to grow so they have been bred with indicas. However, sativa-dominant hybrids provide the patient with the well-known sativa effect. Sativas are useful for a myriad of medical conditions including chronic pain, nausea, depression, some movement disorders, gastrointestinal afflictions, and psychological conditions that benefit from an elevating experience.

Indica

Indica-dominant plants are short squat bushes rather than the Christmas–tree shape of sativas. The fingers of the leaves are shorter and wider too. Indicas form shorter, bulkier, denser, tightly packed oval flowers. Indica-dominant strains have smaller, dense, cone-shaped flowers rather than long cola structures like sativas.

One of indica varieties' medicinal properties is a much deeper body effect than sativa. This semi-lethargic effect makes indicas excellent treatment for deep pains or sleeping disorders. The resinous flowers help patients mentally and physically because of their ability to create a tranquil and carefree feeling. This is helpful for patients with anxiety disorders. Heavily indica-dominant strains should not be used when patients must remain active. They are effective when patients need a more sedative effect. They create a serene feeling that can verge on the spiritual. When taken in large doses the powerful body effects and numbing experience make accomplishing tasks difficult. Some patients find using indica a couple of hours before bedtime helps them sleep for longer periods, rather than having bouts of wakefulness. This deeper rest helps patients feel better and heal faster. Indicas are indicated for conditions where a relaxing, body-focused effect will help. They include movement disorders, bone-joint problems, deep or shooting pains, arthritis, heavy nausea, or other afflictions in which a sedative effect is desired.

Ruderalis

Ruderalis is native to east Europe and the Caucasus. It may be the wild progenitor of sativa and indica subspecies. It has low levels of THC and is not a desirable medicine. Its redeeming quality is the fact that its flowering phase is based chronologically on age, unlike indica or sativa varieties whose flowering is based on the length of the dark period. Breeders crossed ruderalis with sativas and indicas to develop varieties that keep the autoflowering characteristic but retain the THC levels and qualities of indica and sativa strains. The plants usually germinate, grow, and yield ripe flowers in about 100 to 120 days. This makes them ideal for gardening in areas that have a short season. For instance, if the plants were started indoors April 15 and planted outdoors June 1, they would ripen around August 1. Ruderalis hybrids are smaller than other varieties so they are useful for confined spaces.

Hybrids

After years of hybridizing, only a few pure sativa or pure indica landrace strains are available. Most available strains are hybrids of indica and sativa varieties. They carry definitive traits inherited from both sativa and indica progenitors. Hybrids possess the best qualities of both types and offer the most effective genetic combinations. Most hybrids lean one way or another: They are either dominated by the genes of their sativa or indica parents.

Marijuana Varieties

By definition, any marijuana variety can be bred with any other variety to produce a novel plant with distinct genetic characteristics, medicinal properties, and inevitably, a unique name. Most marijuana breeding has taken place in the counterculture. As a result, variety names often seem out-of-place in a medical context. Imagine how difficult it is for some doctors to recommend you try some Granddaddy Purple for your migraine or to seek out a good Trainwreck to increase your appetite. These inappropriate names sometimes deliver unwelcome messages that speak to the illegal black market counterculture, but not to the medical marijuana user. For better or worse these are the common terminologies associated with particular types of marijuana. On the positive side, a patient who has had success using Blue Dream for a particular ailment can go back to their dispensary or provider and ask for that same variety by name with confidence. If you're planting a medical marijuana garden it is best to know that the variety you're growing alleviates your symptoms before you spend months cultivating the crop.

Most varieties have not been developed specifically for medicinal properties. Many were developed to thrive in specific growing conditions or for their high yields. Now that medical cannabis is legal, varieties are bred to target specific medical conditions. For instance, breeders are developing high CBD varieties for patients who require high-CBD/low-THC medicines.

You can consider different varieties of marijuana to be like different flavors. For example, what if you had two favorite flavors and you wanted to combine them to make one super flavor that had the best qualities of both? That super flavor would be a new distinct flavor of its own that

> ## New varieties are constantly bred.

you could call or name whatever you like. Marijuana varieties have been traditionally named this way. Some plants are named for their physical characteristics such as color, aroma, or flavor. The variety Blueberry, bred by DJ Short, smells like blueberries and even has a slightly bluish hue. Sometimes a variety is given a combination of its parents' names to reflect its heritage. For instance, the cross of Blueberry and Trainwreck might be called Bluewreck or Trainberry. Some variety names are even more random or may have a special meaning to the breeder. Marijuana plants have also been named after legendary marijuana activists Jack Herer, Ed Rosenthal, and Lester Grinspoon. New varieties are constantly bred. You may become a strain connoisseur who seeks specific plants or you might find that the particular variety of marijuana you use for treating your symptoms is not important.

Some gardeners are better than others so the quality of the same variety varies. It's important to have a consistent, reliable, trustworthy source to procure the medical marijuana best suited for your own personal needs.

The Spice of Life

The availability of many varieties of marijuana helps both patients and providers. Exploring the therapeutic value of different varieties is the key to deciphering the effectiveness of particular strains for different ailments. As patients become more familiar with the available varieties, researchers will be able to collect more accurate data. If one variety does not work for you, try another. The various chemical combinations of cannabinoids and terpenes (odor molecules) combined with your individual body chemistry create important variables in choosing the right medical marijuana for you. Variety is the spice of life. With medical marijuana, it also enhances your quality of life.

Chapter 7

Growing Marijuana

There are countless ways to grow marijuana. This chapter explores the basic horticultural techniques and provides enough information for you to decide whether you want to pursue growing. If you decide you want to start your own garden, read Ed Rosenthal's *Marijuana Grower's Handbook*, which offers everything you need from garden locations and lighting to choosing varieties.

Marijuana plants are hardy and thrive with the right combination of light, water, air, and grow medium. Provided the right conditions, the plant produces miraculous flowers that are beautiful and very effective in alleviating the symptoms of medical conditions. We'll discuss feeding and maintaining plants, the ideal growing environment, organic growing, and the basics of harvesting, trimming, drying, and curing the crop.

Where to Grow Marijuana

The legal status of marijuana in most of the country drives marijuana cultivators to take extreme measures to conceal their gardens. In states where medical marijuana has some legality patients often are more open about their gardens. Gardeners adapt available spaces to make their gardens in their garage, spare room, attic, closet, basement, garden shed, or a secluded part of the yard. Before choosing a space consider the potential impact on you and the people around you if the garden is seized by authorities and you face legal ramifications. Take security measures to protect the garden from criminals, detection by frenemies, unfriendly neighbors, and law enforcement. Most medical marijuana states allow marijuana gardening as long as you obey local regulations. In these states gardening is far less stressful. However, as long as marijuana remains expensive the threat of criminal activity will remain.

Indoor vs. Outdoor Growing

If you've decided that it's appropriate to grow, your first decision is whether to grow indoors or out. There are, however, distinct differences between growing in a totally controlled indoor environment and gardening outdoors.

Growing Indoors

Indoors, you control the garden environment so you can provide ideal cultivating conditions, in closely modulated light, temperature, nutrients, water, and carbon dioxide. The better the environment, from the plants' point of view, the closer they will come to their full potential and produce a bounteous yield of the highest quality, year-round.

> Whether grown indoors or out, marijuana has similar powerful medical properties and characteristics.

Growing indoors, you avoid exposing the plants to naturally occurring biological contaminants, pests, and weather, which can reduce yield and lower quality and potency. Indoors, you control the weather and light. The light cycle—the length of time the light is on—controls the plants' growth stage: vegetative or flowering. Indoors, you can produce quality flowers several times a year.

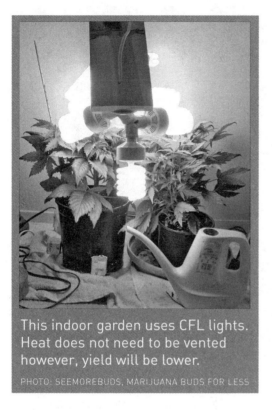
This indoor garden uses CFL lights. Heat does not need to be vented however, yield will be lower.

Another major benefit of indoor gardens is that they are far more difficult to detect. You can keep it hidden from sight, control the odor, and keep unwanted people out. This is especially important in areas with penalties for growing and in neighborhoods with high crime rates.

Growing indoors also has its drawbacks. First, it is expensive. Creating bright light inside isn't cheap. High-wattage lamps, in-line fans, carbon filters, carbon dioxide (CO_2) generators, climate controls like air conditioners and dehumidifiers, pumps, meters, and the electricity it takes to power all this equipment adds up quickly. Another major drawback of indoor growing is the increased risk of property damage from fire, flood, or mold. Proper electrical wiring, adequate ventilation, and rigorous task management make for a safe, productive garden.

Patients may prefer marijuana grown indoors because they believe it is maintained and meticulously harvested to maximize the quantity and offset the high indoor growing cost. Outdoor growers likely have more volume to deal with and thus may pay less attention to details when trimming, curing, and handling the marijuana. For this reason, marijuana grown indoors generally costs more and is seedless.

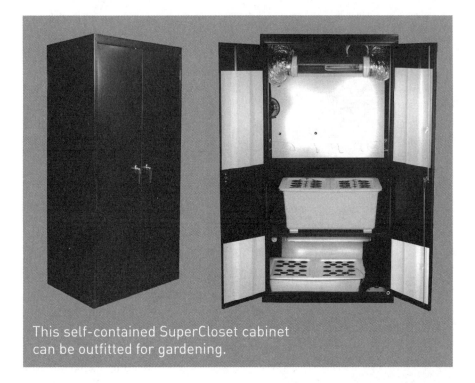

This self-contained SuperCloset cabinet can be outfitted for gardening.

Growing Outdoors

Growing marijuana outdoors has one big advantage: The sun is free. Not only is it free, it is also quite powerful and can create very large marijuana plants. Of course, there is only one growing season outdoors so outdoor growers usually plant their garden in the spring or early summer and harvest it in the fall. The outdoor marijuana crop is susceptible to far more threats than the indoor grow since it is openly exposed to the elements, is more visible, and can more easily become contaminated.

That being said, many marijuana aficionados appreciate the earthy flavorings and complex effects of a well-grown outdoor crop. By avoiding expensive equipment and power bills, an outdoor grower can afford to charge less for the marijuana. If you are lucky enough to live in an area that allows both medical marijuana use and growing medical marijuana outdoors, you may find a relatively inexpensive supply. As the prohibition of medical marijuana is lifted in more states, the prices for marijuana grown outdoors will likely drop considerably.

A drawback to growing outdoors is that you can't control the environment. Your plants are at the mercy of the weather, pests, disease, infection, and inadvertent fertilization by transient pollen from a nearby garden.

Some outdoor gardeners force the plants to flower and ripen early by increasing the dark period each day using tarps or curtains.

Growing in a Greenhouse

Growing marijuana in a greenhouse combines the benefits of using sunlight with the opportunity to control the environment. Greenhouses take advantage of the energy efficiency of the sun while controlling temperature, carbon dioxide (CO_2), humidity, and pests. A greenhouse is a great option, especially in areas with short growing seasons, or susceptibility to unpredictable or harsh weather.

Organic vs. Synthetic Gardening

There is a rising demand for organic foods because organic growers utilize natural fertilizers and avoid chemical pest control. The result is food without chemical residue. The same principles apply to marijuana farming, but no official organic certification programs exist yet. Due to its federal legal status it is impossible to certify organic practices of marijuana production.

There are many synthetic products that work well for growing marijuana including fertilizers, growth additives, and pest control solutions. They may be "completely safe," but they are not organic. Some indoor gardening products meet organic standards. Some outdoor gardening enthusiasts assert that marijuana grown indoors will never be truly organic because of the artificial sunlight factor. This argument is clearly debatable, but indoor gardeners can adhere to organic standards resulting in a natural crop.

Organic Growing

Indoors, organic gardeners usually use an enriched planting mix based on peat moss, bark, or cocoa husk as the growing medium. One popular method is based on feeding the soil and letting the soil feed the plants. Microbes play a roll in breaking down the nutrients. So it takes time to "grow the soil" before growing the plant. Several high quality organic soils are available. Many gardeners amend the mix with natural fertilizers such as bat guano, earthworm castings, and kelp to maintain growth, vitality, and flower production. The movement toward organic production and increased demand for organically grown medical marijuana has led to more availability.

Non-organic/Synthetic

Non-organic methods use mineral fertilizers to maximize yield. Most indoor gardeners produce non-organic plants fed synthetic fertilizer. Synthetic fertilizers and supplements directly feed the plants so they grow very quickly, producing high yields and resulting in medicine with particular desirable characteristics. Hydroponic systems use inert media such as rockwool, clay pellets, or un-enriched planting mix, feeding precise nutrient recipes to produce fast-growing plants. This results in larger, more aromatic, and highly potent flowers that harvest rapidly and possess pharmacologically desired traits.

Some growers use a hybrid of organic and synthetic products. Whether growing organically or non-organically, indoor growers usually "flush" plants with clear water during the final days of flowering to clean out residual fertilizers.

Seed vs. Clone

Plants can be started from seeds or clones. You can plant one seed and hope to get a female plant or you can root a cutting from a female plant and know that your plant is going to grow up female. Indoors, clones are preferred over seeds. Seed companies offer many varieties of "feminized" seeds, which

> One advantage
> of seeds is their
> ease of transport.
> It is easier to
> conceal them
> than to transport
> live plants.

are all-female flowering plants. If you grow from a non-feminized seed, you will need to determine each plant's sex, then remove all the males to eliminate the possibility of pollinating and seeding the females. It is easier to know from the beginning that you have only female plants in your garden, especially if you are growing in a limited space. Seeds are available from companies specializing in them. Most marijuana dispensaries carry a variety of clones for patients.

Growing Mediums

Planting mixes were developed to provide better mediums for indoor gardens. Marijuana also grows well in substrates such as rockwool fiber, clay pellets, coconut husk, perlite, gravel, or un-enriched soil-less mixtures. When using inert media in a hydroponic growing system you control the plant's diet. Whatever substrate you choose, it is important to structure your feeding and watering practices to optimize the medium you've chosen.

Food and Water

Marijuana plants need light, nutrients, CO_2, water, and appropriate temperature and humidity to survive and thrive. The process of getting your plant nutrients and water can make or break a harvest. You can either feed the soil using organic fertilizers and water to dilute these soil components, which will feed the plant, or you can add the nutrients directly into the water and feed the plant through a watering system. Alternatively, you can combine both methods and choose to water fortified soil substrate with nutrient-rich water. Whichever method you choose, in order for the plant to properly take up the nutrients you've provided, the water and feeding solutions must be at the proper pH level. The ideal pH level for marijuana is near 6.0 to 6.3, slightly acidic. The nutrients carried through the water to the roots have to be at an acceptable pH level to be available to the plant. When the pH is right the plants use the nutrients to create growth and produce flowers. Likewise, when the pH is too high or low, the nutrients precipitate and are unavailable to the plant.

Environment

Optimal temperature for growing marijuana is between 75 to 85 degrees during the lit period and 10 degrees colder during the dark period. The ideal humidity range for marijuana is 35 to 55 percent humidity. When it is grown within this range it will grow to its fullest potential. An environment that is too hot, too cold, too dry, or too humid can problems. For instance, a humid environment promotes mold growth. Outdoors, gardeners must adapt their growing methods to their environment.

Trimming, Drying, and Curing

Many people spend three to six months growing a crop and make the big mistake of not taking a few extra days during harvest to trim, dry, and cure the marijuana properly to make it a better product. Hand trimming the leaves of your plants results in an excellent manicure, but can be tedious. There are a number of machines available to assist with trimming larger crops. After trimming it is important to dry the marijuana in a cool, dry place. A temperature between 60 and 70 degrees and a humidity level of 30 to 40 percent is great for drying and curing marijuana. Taking the time to let the buds cure fully enhances the flavor and the bouquet of the medicine and can make it much smoother to consume.

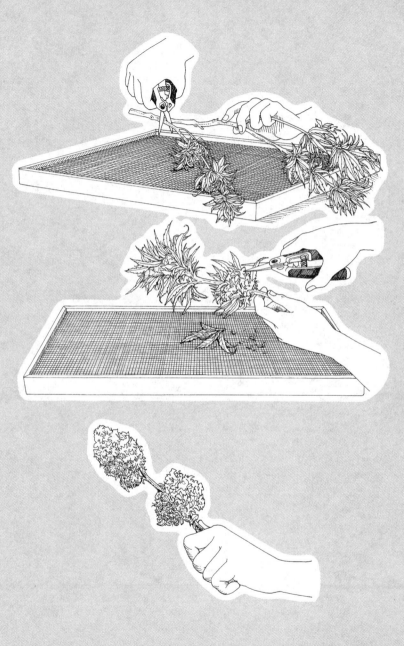

Chapter 8

Your Rights and Responsibilities—
Marijuana Civics and Law

Marijuana laws are rapidly changing and social acceptance for medical marijuana continues to grow. Many patients in need of marijuana have moved to states with more tolerant laws so they can use their medicine without fear of arrest. It's up to you to decide if the reward of treating your condition outweighs the risk of breaking the laws where you live. The most important thing is to avoid ending up in jail for your choice to use marijuana as medicine. An unfortunate encounter with hostile law enforcement can be a life-changing experience. Good people have lost jobs, been put in jail, lost their kids, and been subject to unnecessary ridicule for their choice to relieve their medical symptoms using marijuana.

Know Your Rights

To best way to avoid run-ins with the law while using medical marijuana is to know your rights. Your right to possess, cultivate, or use marijuana varies wildly depending on where you are located. In many states you have no right to use marijuana, period. This doesn't mean you can't use marijuana as a medicine; it means there can be serious consequences if you are caught. Even when medical use is permitted you should be prepared to handle encounters with law enforcement.

If you do intersect with law enforcement don't incriminate yourself or consent to a search. The police may violate your rights even if you assert them. So knowing your rights may not help you avoid a search, arrest, and confiscation of your medicine, but it becomes important in court proceedings. Never consent to a search of your house or property without a properly signed and dated search warrant. Ask the police officer in charge if you are under arrest. If you are not under arrest, ask if you can leave. If you are being arrested, ask to speak to an attorney. Refuse to speak to the police or divulge any information because it can and will be used against you in court. Following these principles can mean the difference between being charged with a serious crime and not being charged at all. If you are a qualified patient with the right to use, possess, or cultivate marijuana, present

---

THE BASICS

- ◎ DON'T CONSENT TO A SEARCH!

- ◎ If the cops say, "Do you mind if I look in your purse, bag, home, or car?"

- ◎ You say, "I do not consent to a search."

- ◎ If cops say, "Why not? Are you hiding something?"

- ◎ You say, "I believe in my Constitutional right to privacy and I do not consent to a search."

- ◎ This probably will not stop an officer from searching you, but it can help get any evidence thrown out in court.

Courtesy of Americans for Safe Access — www.SafeAccessNow.org

---

> If you do intersect with law enforcement don't incriminate yourself or consent to a search.

the proper documentation to the authorities immediately and nothing else. If you are within the boundaries of the law there should be no issue.

Becoming a Qualified Patient

Medical marijuana programs differ from state to state but all require that a doctor or other medical professional approve your use of the medicine. Some states limit the conditions that qualify for use. Others attempt to define the parameters of a doctor-patient relationship claiming the rules prevent abuse or over-prescribing, but their real purpose is to limit patient access. Marijuana is not prescribed because of its federal status as a Schedule I drug, which indicates that it is considered by the authorities to have no medical use. Some states have a medical marijuana patient registry. By getting a recommendation, patients

---

SEARCH WARRANTS

◉ Do NOT let an officer into your home without a search warrant. Check the address, the date—it should be relatively recent—and look for a judge's signature.

◉ If law enforcement knocks on your door, step outside, and close the door behind you while you find out why they are there. Don't leave the door wide open.

◉ If they do enter your home with or without a search warrant say, "I do not consent to a search."

Courtesy of Americans for Safe Access — www.SafeAccessNow.org

can medicate with marijuana without much fear of arrest. In states where medical marijuana use is illegal, patients are not protected from law enforcement. Still having a doctor who is willing to verify your need may be very helpful if legal issues should arise.

The Difference in Federal and State Laws

Some states permit possession, cultivation, and distribution of medical marijuana, but the federal government does not recognize state marijuana laws. As mentioned before, federally, marijuana is a Schedule I controlled substance, meaning it has no formally recognized medicinal value and is illegal to grow, possess, or use. Because of this legal limbo, people who operate legally under state law face prosecution under federal law. Many of these people have been convicted of felonies and sent to prison for growing or providing medical marijuana to legitimate state-certified patients.

MEDICAL MARIJUANA PATIENTS, BE SMART!

Many arrests for marijuana possession are due to traffic violations and noise complaints.

◉ TRAVEL SAFELY: Do not smoke and drive. If you travel with marijuana, make sure your vehicle is up to code and your marijuana is concealed, preferably in your trunk.

◉ BE PREPARED: Carry your doctor's recommendation and state-issued ID card (if you have one) at all times, but do not present it to law enforcement unless accused of a marijuana-related crime.

◉ BE DISCREET: Try not to smoke where others can see you and never leave marijuana items in plain view.

Courtesy of Americans for Safe Access — www.SafeAccessNow.org

---

Navigating Law Enforcement Encounters

If you are a medical marijuana user and intersect with the police, disclose only required or requested information to the officer whether you are a legally qualified patient or not. Even if the police officer is nice, marijuana possession is still a crime so you should never admit guilt. If you are stopped or detained always be respectful of the officer and never pick a fight. You may be totally within your legal rights, but any police officer can make your day more complicated and uncomfortable than it needs to be. Chances are a night in jail won't help your situation medically or otherwise.

If an officer catches you with marijuana or questions you about your use or possession of marijuana, you have a choice to make. You must decide if you will be upfront about your use of medical marijuana or if you will remain silent. Obviously, a big factor in this situation is what the real life consequences are for being in possession of or using marijuana at that given moment and place. If it is minor possession in a fairly liberal area and the cop does not seem overzealous, some would say it may be in your best interest to admit guilt and explain your medical marijuana use. This is not

---

EXERCISE YOUR RIGHTS

There are three levels of police interactions and safe ways to handle each encounter:

◉ 1. CASUAL CONVERSATION: Ask if you are being detained. If not, walk away.

◉ 2. DETENTION: If you are being detained, ask why. Make them cite the law and remember what they say.

◉ 3. ARRESTS: Say, "I choose to remain silent and want to speak to a lawyer." Remember to remain silent.

Courtesy of Americans for Safe Access — www.SafeAccessNow.org

If you are growing marijuana it is important to stay within the allotted guidelines and follow the letter of the law.

usually the case. Never admit that you were involved in "criminal" activity, no matter how tempting it might seem. If you are in a state where medical marijuana is allowed and you are within the boundaries of the prevailing local and state laws, you should have no issue disclosing you are in possession of or using marijuana within your legal rights. If you are in a hostile environment, however, or you feel the officer has a bias against marijuana and wants to take you to jail, your best bet is to remain silent and ask if you are being arrested. If you're not being arrested, ask if you can leave and be on your way immediately or as soon as possible. If an officer wants to search your home, car, or person without cause, exercise your right to privacy and do not consent to the search. Chances are they may search anyway; but you have at least expressed your non-consent, which will help you in court.

If you are growing marijuana it is important to stay within the allotted guidelines and follow the letter of the law. The police want to find you out of compliance so they can hassle you, which they feel is part of their job. Cultivating marijuana illegally generally carries much steeper penalties than simple possession, so it is important to understand and exercise your rights. You should investigate the laws regarding illegal gardens where you live. If you choose to grow a medical garden in an area where it is not allowed be sure to have a local attorney available should an issue arise.

Be Safe or Be Sorry

Many patients have experiences with the law because they failed to adhere to some basic safety principles.

- Avoid telling people about your private use or medical marijuana cultivation. Often people are detected or turned over to law enforcement by others after they bragged about their garden to a person who told another person and so on. You can remain safe by not disclosing your marijuana use, possession, or cultivation.

- Never use marijuana and put yourself in a dangerous situation, such as operating heavy or dangerous machinery. Legal issues can arise for both patient and caregiver if medical marijuana is used irresponsibly.

- Never steal electricity when cultivating.

- Growers must not overload electrical circuits. It is unwise and unsafe because it can cause a fire. Make sure all wiring is up to code. Always be safe, not sorry.

Chapter 9

The Marijuana Industry

In states where the medical marijuana industry has blossomed, jobs are being created, taxes are being paid, and thriving new businesses are making a positive impact on local economies. In comparison, the prohibition of marijuana has created a black market. Consequently the government continues to spend over $30 billion a year arresting, prosecuting, and punishing marijuana users. The quasi-legal status of marijuana keeps consumer prices high because of continued risk to suppliers. As the legal market emerges, supply and demand will dictate consumer prices.

As safe access to medical marijuana becomes widely available, a larger segment of the population will be able to access cannabinoid-based therapies. When normalized, patients will feel more comfortable using the medicine so the market will continue to grow. The industry is still developing. However, until marijuana is fully legalized for medical use the industry will not reach its full economic potential.

A Penny Saved

It costs a lot of money to employ law enforcement to arrest, attorneys to prosecute, and for the prison union lobby to incarcerate the country's medical marijuana users. Green Aid, The Medical Marijuana Legal Defense and

Education Fund, estimates that federal and state governments spend over $30 billion dollars each year arresting and prosecuting marijuana users including many medical marijuana users.

Not So Niche a Market

Medical marijuana patients come from many different walks of life: the successful businessman, notable senior citizen, thriving college student, local car salesman, and soccer mom. You may be surprised at who is a medical marijuana patient. Your neighbor, the checker at the grocery store, or a person at your work could have a condition that marijuana benefits. A CNN/ *Time* poll from October 2002 revealed 80 percent of Americans, "think adults should be allowed to legally use marijuana for medical purposes if their doctor prescribes it." Illness touches every corner of our communities, so it is incorrect to classify marijuana as a "niche" or "limited" market. Marijuana is mainstream and more people use it every day. This is creating a larger demand and as a result a more professional industry is developing to meet it.

CannaBusiness

One interesting aspect of the marijuana industry is seeing the once clandestine marijuana producer develop a legal tax-paying business. There is a growing desire for marijuana providers to be accepted as normal members of the community. However, some local governments, at the behest of the criminal justice system, have imposed unnecessarily strict regulations, levied hefty taxes, and been critical of marijuana-related businesses. Some local jurisdictions have imposed onerous zoning regulations on dispensaries and other marijuana businesses. Some of these are much more stringent than regulations imposed on liquor stores and sexually oriented businesses. These regulations make it far more difficult and expensive to operate, resulting in higher prices for patients. This is a transfer of wealth from sick patients to the state, unlike other pharmaceuticals, which are sold free of sales taxes.

Even with the risks and hurdles that still exist, the movement toward business-minded principles and practices continues. What were once rogue, fringe marijuana "clubs" have evolved into well-respected medical dispensaries. These specialty businesses pepper the landscape in states that permit them and have become a model for legal marijuana distribution. Medical marijuana states have developed a number of different models to regulate distribution outlets. For instance, some states require that dispensaries be not-for-profit organizations.

Government Revenues

The commercialization of medical marijuana through dispensaries benefits local economies and state and local government revenues. Rather than a "nuisance" issue for local governments, medical marijuana is an economic dynamo. The California State Board of Equalization estimates that over $100 million in tax revenue is paid on the sale of medical marijuana every year. In 2010 Colorado collected $7.34 million just in application fees for medical marijuana businesses. These revenues are only part of the picture. The sales tax is an indication of total sales. People employed throughout the chain include growers, manicurists, dispensary buyers, packagers, retail clerks—and all of the employees associated with running a business. In California more than 100,000 people earn a living from medical marijuana.

In the midst of a stark economic downturn and crumbling infrastructure, the

> Even with the risks and hurdles that still exist, the movement toward business-minded principles and practices continues.

thriving marijuana industry is gaining rapid fiscal acceptance. Even extremely conservative communities are beginning to accept the medical marijuana industry. Some areas have imposed higher than normal rates of taxation on medical marijuana businesses. Patients bear the brunt of the taxation with higher prices. This "pay-to-play" situation is less than ideal for the marijuana patient. This is an unfair tax on sick people for obtaining safe medicines and results in a transfer of wealth from the sick to the state.

Supporting Industries

In addition to businesses that directly provide medicine to patients, an array of associated industries sprouted up to meet the unique needs of the medical marijuana community.

Gardeners want to optimize their production and are willing to spend more than farmers for most crops. Many specialty products are available to enhance yield and quality. Indoor gardeners often use high-tech equipment costing thousands of dollars. There is keen competition between brands of lights, fertilizers, growing mediums, environmental monitors and controls, security systems, and odor-control units. Outdoor gardeners purchase soil amendments, fertilizers, and other plant maintenance equipment. During harvest season in traditional marijuana growing communities like Humboldt County in Northern California, major retailers stock trays, storage containers, trimming scissors, and other items used for manicuring crops. Some growers hire cooks or caterers to feed the manicurists, also known as trimmers.

Doctors who specialize in marijuana referrals also thrive. Dr. Tod Mikuriya opened the first full-time marijuana consultation clinic in California shortly after the passage of the Compassionate Use Act of 1996. Many doctors are unwilling to recommend marijuana to patients so physicians who are willing to provide medical marijuana recommendations have developed this specialty. In most states, recommendations are updated annually so hundreds of thousands of patients require recommendations every year. Medical professionals keep up-to-date recommendations as an insurance policy against incarceration.

Quality control is also emerging as a growth industry. Analytical laboratories test for contaminants and levels of THC, CBD, and other cannabinoids. The DEA imposes restrictions on registered labs, making it impossible for them to perform these tests for growers and dispensaries. Marijuana-specific laboratories fill the void. These services increase the amount of information available to patients, helping them make informed purchasing decisions.

Marijuana businesses employ consultants, accountants, and attorneys. Industry-specific publications provide information to patients and dispensary owners.

The market for pipes and vaporizers is increasing. Decorative glass pipes, innovative vaporizers, and lab-glass quality waterpipes are sold in

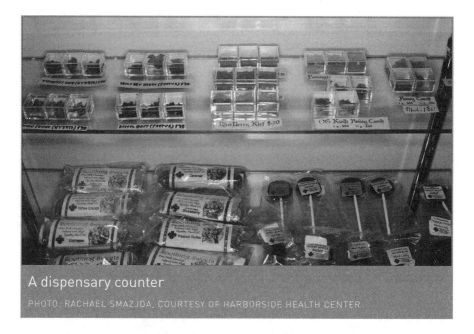

A dispensary counter

stores and on Web sites that specialize solely in marijuana smoking-related gear. There are also multitudes of other products targeted to medical marijuana users: drug-test-masking agents, clothing, music, and novelty goods.

The many associated industries that support and cater to the medical marijuana industry continue to grow rapidly. There are marijuana-inspired eateries, such as Chronic Tacos in California and Cheeba Hut in Colorado that overtly market to marijuana users. As patient demand has risen, providers, producers, and businesses are there to provide the goods.

Marijuana Jobs

Fact: The marijuana industry creates jobs. Producers of marijuana employ people with various skills to tend to the gardens, harvest, and trim the crop. Delivery services and private caregivers are paid to provide marijuana and related care to patients. As mentioned earlier, some doctors specialize in

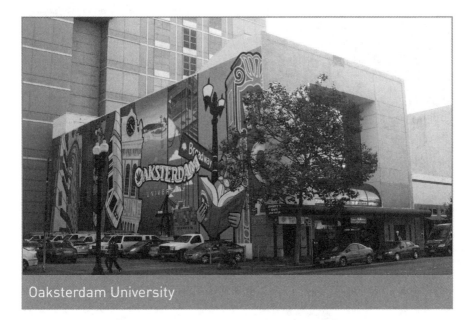

Oaksterdam University

recommending marijuana. They employ receptionists, nurses, accountants, and assistants. We also noted that dispensaries employ extensive staffs, including managers, buyers, security guards, service staff, transporters, and "bud tenders."

A "bud tender" is the term for a patient-care specialist who handles and dispenses marijuana, much like a pharmacy technician. A "buyer" or vendor coordinator evaluates and purchases marijuana and other cannabis products for the dispensary. The industry has created numerous, previously unheard of, specialty positions that provide job security. Several trade schools and "universities" provide training, knowledge, and support for those wishing to enter the industry.

Fact: The marijuana industry creates jobs.

Marijuana is used to prepare medical ingestibles and many people are involved in food production and preparation. Unions are recruiting members from dispensaries and other marijuana-related businesses. Several trade associations have formed to represent the industry and give it a lobbying voice. The industry is expanding and as it does, the number of people finding stable and secure employment in producing and distributing medical marijuana is increasing. Over 100,000 people are involved directly in the marijuana supply chain and over 250,000 earn their living from marijuana-related businesses.

Chapter 10

The Future of Medical Marijuana

No one can say for certain what the future holds for medical marijuana. What seems certain is the toothpaste is out of the tube and it will be extremely difficult to put it back in. Return to complete prohibition and repeal of liberalized state laws on medical marijuana seems highly unlikely. Over time as the sky does not fall, the world does not end, and increasing numbers of constituents benefit from the more enlightened laws, perhaps the political charades surrounding marijuana will cease and our lawmakers will advance the cause by allowing more active research and medical implementation. As positive research findings continue to be released and the benefits of medical marijuana are revealed, word will spread. Until then, we must engage our friends and neighbors in honest conversations about medical marijuana use and the patients who get relief from it.

It is fascinating to ponder the possibilities inherent to the resurgence of medical marijuana. Scientists, are unlocking the secrets of why different varieties of marijuana work best for different conditions. It is exciting to witness the industry's evolution from the underground to part of the regular economy.

Appendix I
Big Pharma vs. the Small Organic Grower

Not since the dot-com bubble of the late '90s has there been as much buzz about a developing industry and its growth potential. As more people begin to use marijuana medically, calls for reform continue. One of the big questions is how pharmaceutical companies will respond as marijuana becomes a legal medicine. Marijuana is a plant that almost anybody can grow regardless of skill, location, or socioeconomic status. Large drug manufacturing companies are conducting research into its uses and they will produce cannabinoid-based medicines. The medicines they will produce will most likely be derivatives of marijuana, or synthetics based on its chemistry, not a botanical form. There will still be a demand for high quality herbal medicines that farmers and growers are sure to supply.

Appendix II

Research and Development

As research and development continue, mysteries of how the marijuana plant interacts with the body's receptors will lead to medical breakthroughs. Through genetic mapping, cannabinoid profiling, and clinical trials performed in the finest U.S. scientific laboratories and universities, we will begin to understand why this plant is so beneficial. Patients will benefit from the growing specialization in the areas of symptom control and condition-based treatment determined by using specific genetic profiles and different qualities of the countless strains of marijuana available. We will gain a greater understanding of the properties of cannabinoids and terpenes. Many scientists are already exploring possibilities in this uncharted territory. With more research, medical marijuana may become a key that unlocks the door to the comfort and wellness of humankind.

Appendix III
Medical Marijuana Now

There's too much political noise in the medical marijuana argument. The legal, appropriate use of medical marijuana should be a given. It is unconscionable to think that politicians can stand in the way of a single person's health. Drug reform is an uphill battle but we are changing the laws and are protecting more patients with each passing day. Instead of turning a blind eye or making excuses, it is time for public officials to develop reasonable regulations allowing patients to use medical marijuana. Anything less is uncivilized.

BIBLIOGRAPHY
(in order of reference)

The Marihuana Tax Act of 1937, Full text with commentary. The Shaffer Library of Drug Policy.

http://www.druglibrary.org/schaffer/History/HISTORY.HTM

Controlled Substances Act of 1970 and Latest Current Version. U.S. Drug Enforcement Administration.

http://www.justice.gov/dea/pubs/csa.html

American Medical Association. "Support of Rescheduling of Marijuana Report 3" of the Council on Science and Public Health (I-09), "Use of Cannabis for Medicinal Purposes" (Resolutions 910, I-08; 921, I-08; and 229, A-09), 2010.

http://www.ama-assn.org/resources/doc/csaph/csaph-report3-i09.pdf

American College of Physicians. "Supporting Research into the Therapeutic Role of Marijuana," 2008.

http://www.acponline.org/advocacy/where_we_stand/other_issues/medmarijuana.pdf

American Public Health Association Resolution 9513: "Access to Therapeutic Marijuana/Cannabis," 1995.

http://www.drugpolicy.org/docUploads/APHAendorse.pdf

National Institute of Drug Abuse, U.S. Department of Health and Human Services. Research Monograph 44: "Marijuana Effects on the Endocrine and Reproductive Systems," 1983.

http://archives.drugabuse.gov/pdf/monographs/44.pdf

Cannabis International—A resource for the dietary and medicinal study and use of cannabis. Website contains hundreds of research articles, interviews and lists of resources.

http://cannabisinternational.org

"Reefer Madness: Marijuana Is Medically Useful Whether Politicians Like It or Not," *The Economist*, April 27, 2008.

Steep Hill Cannabis Analysis Laboratory, Oakland, California.

www.steephilllab.com

"Respiratory symptoms and lung function in habitual heavy smokers of marijuana alone, smokers of marijuana and tobacco, smokers of tobacco alone, and nonsmokers" by DP Tashkin, AH Coulson, VA Clark et al. *American Journal of Respiratory and Critical Care Medicine*: 135(1), 209–216, 1987.

Patients Out of Time— A compassionate, science-based educational forum for the restoration of medical cannabis knowledge.

www.MedicalCannabis.com

Center for Medical Cannabis Research at University of California, San Diego.

www.cmcr.ucsd.edu/

Americans for Safe Access—Advancing Legal Marijuana Therapeutics and Research.

www.AmericansForSafeAccess.org

Colorado Medical Marijuana Enforcement Rules.

http://www.colorado.gov/cs/Satellite/Rev-Enforcement/
RE/1251575119584

Wo/Men's Alliance for Medical Marijuana (WAMM)—A Collective of Patients and Caregivers, Santa Cruz, CA.

www.wamm.org

"Large Study Finds No Link between Marijuana and Lung Cancer" by David Biello, *Scientific American*, May 24, 2006.

The Big Book of Buds Volume 4: Marijuana Varieties from the World's Great Seed Breeders by Ed Rosenthal. Quick American, 2010.

Marijuana Grower's Handbook by Ed Rosenthal. Quick American, 2010.

Suggested Further Reading

Aunt Sandy's Medical Marijuana Cookbook by Sandy Moriarty. Quick American Archives, 2010

Marihuana: The First Twelve Thousand Years by Ernest L. Abel. McGraw-Hill, 1982

Marihuana: The Forbidden Medicine by Dr. Lester Grinspoon M.D. and Dr. James B. Bakalar , 1997

Marijuana Grower's Handbook: Official Coursebook of Oaksterdam University by Ed Rosenthal. Foreword by Tommy Chong. Quick American Archives, 2010

Marijuana Medical Handbook: Practical Guide to Therapeutic Uses of Marijuana by Ed Rosenthal, Dale Gieringer Ph.D., and Dr. Tod Mikuriya M.D. Quick American Archives, 1996

Marijuana: Medical Papers, 1839-1972 (Cannabis: Collected Clinical Papers) by Tod H. Mikuriya M.D. Symposium Press, 2007